☽ Get
a
Good Night's
Sleep ☾

Katherine A. Albert, M.D., Ph.D.

A FIRESIDE BOOK
Published by Simon & Schuster

F

FIRESIDE
Rockefeller Center
1230 Avenue of the Americas
New York, NY 10020

First Fireside Edition 1997

FIRESIDE and colophon are registered trademarks
of Simon & Schuster Inc.

Designed by Monika Keano, *Studio Bird*

Manufactured in the United States of America

10 9 8 7 6 5 4 3 2 1

Library of Congress Cataloging-in-Publication Data
Albert, Katherine A.
    Get a good night's sleep/Katherine A. Albert
        p. cm.
    1. Insomnia.   I. Title.
RC548. A43   1996
616.8'498—dc20   96-21034   CIP

ISBN 0-684-80428-X
       0-684-83527-4 (Pbk)

The ideas, procedures, and suggestions in this book are not
intended as a substitute for the medical advice of a trained
health professional. All matters regarding your health require
medical supervision. Consult your physician before adopting
the suggestions in this book, as well as about any condition
that may require diagnosis or medical attention. The authors
and the publisher disclaim any liability arising directly or
indirectly from the use of techniques in this book.

ACKNOWLEDGMENTS

Many thanks go to Betsy Ryan, president of Bascom Communications, who produced this book with intelligence and care. My gratitude goes also to Rachel Kranz, a gifted writer; Bob Bender, my talented editor; and peerless Johanna Li.

For Emma and Hugh

CONTENTS

. . . sleep is the golden chain that ties health and our bodies together.

—Thomas Dekker (1572–1632)

) Get
a
Good Night's

Sleep (

Chapter 1

How Common Is Insomnia?

Now, blessings light on him that first invented sleep! It covers a man all over, thoughts and all, like a cloak; it is meat for the hungry, drink for the thirsty, heat for the cold, and cold for the hot. It is the current coin that purchases all the pleasures of the world cheap, and the balance that sets the king and the shepherd, the fool and the wise man, even.

—Cervantes, *Don Quixote*

Falling asleep seems like the simplest task—until you can't do it. One sleepless night seems to deprive you of the pleasures of resting, of dreaming, of escaping from the world for a little while and returning refreshed and energized. Lying awake, tossing and turning, perhaps alone, perhaps with a peacefully sleeping partner nearby, can feel lonely, frustrating, depressing—and exhausting. Maybe the worst part is the growing sense of anxiety, the fear that an act once so easily accomplished is now forever out of reach. In your desperate thirst for sleep, you begin to worry that you'll never fall asleep again.

If this description of insomnia sounds familiar to you, take heart. You're not alone—and there is help. Sorting through the myths and facts about sleep and sleeplessness can help you figure out why sleep is eluding you and what you can do to recover it. Learning more about the biology of sleep, as well as about your own habits, can put you on the road to more frequent sleep-filled nights followed by mornings when you feel well rested and energized. Better still, as you learn more about sleep—and about yourself—you might even be able to improve your sleep, spending fewer hours in bed while feeling more rested. Part of the problem with trying to address insomnia is the number of myths that people have about sleep. Often the very things they do to bring sleep closer actually push sleep further away. How much do you know about sleep? Take the following quiz and find out.

MYTHS AND FACTS ABOUT SLEEP AND SLEEPLESSNESS

Choose the correct answer from among the given choices.

1. You're waking up feeling tired and groggy. Which of the following is most likely to help you feel more rested?
  a. sleeping more hours
  b. sleeping fewer hours
  c. making sure you get more sleep before midnight
  d. getting more sleep on the weekends

2. Tomorrow morning, you have to get up three hours earlier than usual to catch an early plane. The best way for you to stay rested is to
  a. take a nap the afternoon *after* your early morning.
  b. take a nap the afternoon *before* your early morning.
  c. go to bed three hours earlier.
  d. get three hours more sleep the next night.

3. You've been having trouble falling asleep, and a friend suggests getting more exercise. The most sleep-inducing time to exercise is

    a. right before bedtime.

    b. two hours before bedtime.

    c. several hours before bedtime.

    d. first thing in the morning.

4. If you lose a night of sleep, in order to make up for it you need

    a. eight extra hours of sleep.

    b. six extra hours of sleep.

    c. four extra hours of sleep.

    d. two extra hours of sleep.

5. If you're feeling sleepy during the day and you want to perk yourself up, the best thing you can drink at lunch is

    a. a cup of coffee.

    b. a glass of skim milk.

    c. a cola drink.

    d. a cup of herb tea.

Decide whether each statement is true or false.

___ **6.** A person is born with a definite need for a certain number of hours of sleep.

___ **7.** A healthy person needs at least eight hours of sleep.

___ **8.** Everyone is born either a "night owl" or a "lark," and there is very little anyone can do to change his or her pattern.

___ **9.** Sleep is important because that's when your body and your mind "turn off," relax, and do virtually nothing.

___ **10.** A person's "natural" biological clock runs on a twenty-four-hour cycle, so, left to ourselves, we would always go to sleep and get up at regular hours.

How did you do? Take a look at the answers, and see if you've been operating on incorrect assumptions about sleep and sleeplessness.

1. You're waking up feeling tired and groggy. Which of the following is most likely to help you feel more rested?
   a. *sleeping more hours*
   b. *sleeping fewer hours*
   c. making sure you get more sleep before midnight
   d. getting more sleep on the weekends

Most people assume that tiredness is caused by lack of sleep—and it may be. But sometimes, tiredness is also caused by spending *too much time in bed.* Ironically, you might actually feel more rested if you spend less time in bed, especially if you improve your sleep hygiene in some of the other ways discussed later in this book.

When a person sleeps—before or after midnight, at night or during the day—is not necessarily related to feeling tired or not, although some people may find that their lives work better with earlier or later bedtimes. Getting more sleep on the weekends is probably the worst way of recovering from exhaustion, since an irregular schedule is the most tiring of all. (For more about schedules and sleep, see Chapter 5.)

2. Tomorrow morning, you have to get up three hours earlier than usual to catch an early plane. The best way for you to stay rested is to

    a. *take a nap the afternoon* after *your early morning.*
    b. take a nap the afternoon before your early
       morning.
    c. go to bed three hours earlier.
    d. get three hours more sleep the next night.

Your body responds least well to varying your sleep schedule—so going to bed at your usual time, even if you're getting up early, will probably be more restful for you in the long run. For the same reason, keeping your usual wake-up time is also a good idea, which is why a nap is better than sleeping longer the next night. You will not be able to sleep the afternoon before unless you are sleep deprived.

    3. You've been having trouble falling asleep, and a friend suggests getting more exercise. The most sleep-inducing time to exercise is
    a. right before bedtime.
    b. two hours before bedtime.
    c. *several hours before bedtime.*
    d. first thing in the morning.

Generally, exercise is helpful to overcoming sleep problems—but exercise also raises your body temperature, which wakes you up. Exercising at the end of the day—after your workday and before your evening meal—is probably your most sleep-inducing choice, because the exercise is a great way to release the accumulated stress of the workday while decreasing your appetite for dinner, helping you to stick to the light supper that most sleep experts recommend. (For more on the relationship between food and sleep, see

Chapter 4.) Exercising first thing in the morning may also be a good choice, as many people find that this helps them to wake up. Exercising too close to bedtime, however, will make you feel more wakeful for a while, which is counterproductive if you've been having trouble falling asleep. (For more on exercise and sleep, see Chapter 6.)

4. If you lose a night of sleep, in order to make up for it you need

    a. eight extra hours of sleep.

    b. six extra hours of sleep.

    c. four extra hours of sleep.

    d. two extra hours of sleep.

If you lose only one night of sleep, you only need approximately 25 percent of the missing sleep to make up your lost rest. For most people, that will amount to two hours or less to recuperate one lost night. By the same token, if you miss two full nights of sleep in a row, you can make it up with no more than four extra hours. People who have been artificially sleep-deprived for several days in laboratory tests are able to make up their lost sleep in several hours, with no apparent long-lasting ill effects. However, chronic sleep deprivation can require six weeks of as much sleep as one needs before all of the ill effects are reversed.

5. If you're feeling sleepy during the day and you want to perk yourself up, the best thing you can drink at lunch is

    a. a cup of coffee.

    b. a glass of skim milk.

c. a cola drink.
d. *a cup of herb tea.*

Although most people turn to coffee or cola for the stimulating effects of caffeine, they are likely to find that the lift is soon followed by a crash. Even if the coffee-drinker is one of those people who continues to feel the effects of caffeine for twelve to twenty hours after ingesting it, he or she may feel both wired and tired. If the cola drink has sugar in it, that might also perk someone up for a while, but the sugar high will soon lead to a sugar low.

Some people may find that the protein in a glass of milk gives them a midafternoon lift, especially when there's no fat in the milk to burden their digestions. However, milk contains tryptophan, a natural relaxant, which could actually make a person feel sleepier. (That's why a glass of warm milk is often a good before-bedtime drink—unless the milk drinker is one of the many people who is lactose-intolerant or has some other kind of allergy to milk.) Therefore, the best daytime pick-me-up drink is some kind of sugar-free, caffeine-free, tryptophan-free beverage—like herb tea.

6. A person is born with a definite need for a certain number of hours of sleep. *True.*

While our need for sleep is highest in infancy and then decreases to a certain adult level, that adult level is biologically determined and is different for different people. However, this need for sleep may vary in a minor way over time. What we eat and when, how much we exercise and when, how much stress is going on in our lives, and a host of other factors, influence how much sleep we need, as well as the quality of the sleep we get. (For more about the different factors that affect your need for sleep, see Chapter 2.)

7. A healthy person needs at least eight hours of sleep. *False.*

Just as individual needs for food vary, so do individual needs for sleep. Although most people seem to need between six and nine hours of sleep each night, some people seem to do quite well on four or five, while others need ten. And, as mentioned above, the amount of sleep that any person needs can vary somewhat, depending on the person's lifestyle, state of mind, and beliefs about sleep.

8. Everyone is born either a "night owl" or a "lark," and there is very little that anyone can do to change his or her pattern. *False.*

Most people have no strong owl or lark tendencies. However, research does show that about 20 percent of the population is biologically "wired" in one direction or the other. The other 80 percent can adapt with some effort to whatever schedule demands come their way—although it seems to take about three weeks for people to adapt to extreme changes, such as starting a night shift or getting up two or three hours earlier.

9. Sleep is important because that's when your body and your mind "turn off," relax, and do virtually nothing. *False.*

In fact, our minds and our bodies are both quite active during sleep, and bodily restoration and repair take place around the clock, although these functions peak and fall according to various cycles. Basically, though, no scientist can explain with any certainty exactly why our bodies seem to need sleep. (For more on the biological nature of sleep, see Chapter 2.)

Actually, most sleep experts are somewhat baffled by the topic they study. They don't really know *why* we need to sleep—only that everybody does. Sleep seems to have both a psychological function—connected to dreaming—and a physiological function, although even this basic formulation has been debated and disputed by scientists from different disciplines. The latest research suggests that our physical need for sleep seems related to maintaining our immune system.

10. A person's "natural" biological clock runs on a twenty-four-hour cycle, so, left to ourselves, we would always go to sleep and get up at regular hours. *False.*

In fact, although the earth spins on a twenty-four-hour cycle, our bodies are more comfortable running at twenty-four and a half or even twenty five. And experiments done on people deprived of information about what time it is or whether it is day or night have discovered that people's cycles seem rather free-running. Left to themselves, people might stay up for twenty hours or more at a time and then sleep for ten or twelve hours. In order to accommodate ourselves to the earth's twenty-four-hour rotation and our civilization's eight-hour day, we seem to require a lot of external cues. On the other hand, people who—like most of us—do have to live on the world's schedule seem to do better with regular sleeping and waking times. That's why establishing a bedtime routine is often such a good idea, especially for people with sleeping problems. (For more about bedtime routines, see Chapter 7.)

You Are Not Alone!

For the vast majority of Americans, sleep disorders represent another silent epidemic, much as hypertension was characterized a decade ago. Neither the public nor their physicians understand that sleep disorders [such as insomnia, narcolepsy, and sleep apnea] are real illnesses with serious and pernicious effects or that such disorders are susceptible to intervention. Unfortunately . . . no existing program is responsible for general public awareness about the importance of sleep hygiene, the risks of inadequate rest, or the recognition of a sleep problem as a symptom of a mental disorder.

—from "Wake Up America: A National Sleep Alert," September 1992 report by the National Committee on Sleep Disorders Research to Congress and the U.S. Department of Health and Human Services

When you're tossing and turning at three in the morning, unable to fall into sleep, it may *seem* as though you alone are being denied the delights of slumber. In fact, many insomniacs have complained about the sense of loneliness and isolation as one of the worst side effects of their condition. However, the truth is, you are far from alone in your sleepless state. Scientists have estimated that some 100 million Americans suffer from some form of insomnia—difficulty in initiating or maintaining sleep. An estimated 20 million Americans suffer from *chronic* insomnia—sleep problems that persist for more than three weeks—and of these, some 70 percent seek help, often from one of the more than 250 accredited sleep centers located across the country, or from the thousand or more somnologists who specialize in treating sleep disorders.

More specific studies reveal that the problem may be even more widespread. A study of one thousand households in Los Angeles found that one-third of the families inter-viewed included someone who was currently having problems with insomnia, while 42 percent contained a member who had had difficulties with sleep at one time. A Gallup poll con-ducted for *Esquire* magazine found that 50 percent of the re-spondents had trouble falling asleep or staying awake. A study undertaken in Gainesville, Florida, by psychiatrist Ismet Karacan, comprising 1,645 people, discovered that one-third to one-half had trouble sleeping. And in a survey of some three thousand doctors in a range of specialties—including surgery, neurology, and obstetrics/gynecology—found that al-most 19 percent of their patients complained of various forms of insomnia. In fact, according to one expert, more people complain to their doctors about not getting enough sleep than about any other complaint.

Insomnia is an extremely uncomfortable and frustrat-ing condition for those who suffer from it—but the costs don't stop there. Some estimates place insomnia's cost to the nation as high as $70 billion in lost productivity, medical bills, and accidents. The sleeplessness of doctors, pilots, and some engineers places numerous people in jeopardy. Sleep problems also dangerously diminish the efficiency of sewage-treatment plant operators and workers at nuclear power plants. Studies in Oklahoma and California found that the driver's sleepiness was a factor in about 20 percent of all highway accidents.

Sleep-related disorders are a special problem for shift workers—those whose jobs require something other than a nine-to-five schedule, and particularly those whose jobs require rotating schedules. Over 13 million Americans—approximately 20 percent of the workforce—work full- or part-time jobs in the evenings or at night. Even if their job schedules do not rotate, they are likely to live on a night schedule during the work week and a day schedule on their days off, causing particular difficulties with sleeping. One plant estimated that 76 percent of their workers had trouble sleeping; another study found that half of all shift workers fell asleep on their job at least once a week, while 15 percent fell asleep at the wheel of a car at least once every three months. Workers on unusual shifts average five more absent days per year, and they are more likely than others to become dependent on caffeine, drugs, alcohol, and over-the-counter sleep aids and stimulants. At one plant, a study found that two-thirds of the workers took an alcoholic drink at bedtime at least once a week, while some 12 percent relied on sleeping pills.

The Other Side of the Coin: Subjective Insomnia

> How many thousands of my poorest subjects
> Are at this hour asleep!
> O sleep, O gentle sleep,
> Nature's soft nurse, how have I frighted thee,
> That thou no more wilt weigh my eyelids down
> And steep my sense in forgetfulness?
>
> —Shakespeare, *Henry IV,* Part I

The restless king in Shakespeare's play believes that sleep has deserted him—but a modern sleep specialist might consider the possibility that Henry is getting more sleep than he realizes. Although insomnia is a very real problem, researchers speak of an equally real problem known as *subjective insomnia*. People with subjective insomnia believe that they are sleeping far less than is actually the case.

Spouses may attest to subjective insomnia in their sleeping partners. A bed partner may notice that his or her mate seemed to sleep soundly for much of the night—even to the point of waking the sleeping partner with his or her loud snores! Yet the next morning, the sleeper attests that he or she "didn't sleep a wink," "was up all night," or "barely slept."

Sleep clinics support the perception that many self-described insomniacs may be getting more sleep than they realize. Sleep clinics specialize in diagnosing and treating sleep disorders such as insomnia. Most causes of insomnia can be treated without recording the patient's sleep. If however, after thorough consultation, there is no clear diagnosis, they may invite the patient to spend a night in the sleep laboratory, hooked up to a range of electrodes and sensors that monitor their sleep-wake patterns, the various types of sleep and dreaming activity that go on during their sleep, and other biological functions such as heart rate, respiratory activity, eye movements, and muscle tension. We can assume that if anyone has an objective picture of a person's sleep patterns, it would be a clinical observer. Indeed, if anything, a patient is likely to sleep *less* well in the unfamiliar clinic than at home in his or her own bed. Yet sleep clinics report that half of all people who say they can't sleep only *think* they can't.

This perception was confirmed by a study conducted at the University of Chicago in which two people with mild insomnia were compared with thirty-two who had normal sleep patterns. Although the insomniacs told researchers that it took them an average of one hour to fall asleep, laboratory researchers found that it actually took them only fifteen minutes—a completely normal amount of time. (In fact, if you're falling asleep in much less than ten or fifteen minutes, it may be a sign that you're sleep-deprived.) Researchers did find that the self-described insomniacs awoke more often than the normal sleepers, but laboratory instruments showed that this made for relatively little difference in total sleep time: five and three-quarters hours for the insomniacs versus six and a half hours for the normal sleepers.

Why do people get subjective insomnia? In some cases, they're simply not aware of how long it takes people to fall asleep. Although, as we've seen, it takes a normally rested person ten to fifteen minutes, many of us believe that we should fall asleep "as soon as my head hits the pillow." When that doesn't happen, we feel cheated, frustrated, or perhaps inadequate, especially if a sleeping partner manages to fall asleep more quickly than we do.

In other cases, people misinterpret their own sleep patterns. It's a little-known fact that most people wake frequently during the night, especially as they get older. That's why we're able to remember our dreams—we often wake briefly after a particularly vivid, exciting, or troubling dream, often without fully realizing that we *are* awake—and then fall quickly back to sleep. A person who believes he or she has insomnia may take somewhat longer to fall asleep. He or she may remember only the wakefulness, forgetting the periods of sleep in between.

Dreams may also affect our perceptions of sleep. Some people dream that they're awake and then remember the dream. Others sleep lightly and have the sense that they're aware of the world around them, even though clinically their brains are functioning in a sleeping, not a waking, state.

If you're wondering whether you, too, have subjective insomnia, you don't necessarily have to go to a sleep clinic to find out. Here's a simple alternative: Put a pencil and notebook within easy reach of your bed. As the thought occurs to you, glance at the clock and write down the time. In the morning, you may be surprised to find that the intervals between time entries suddenly go from ten and fifteen minutes to several hours.

Of course, even if subjective insomniacs are getting more sleep than they thought, they might not be getting as much sleep as they need. Everyone's sleep needs are different, and each of our needs varies at different times of our lives, depending on our age, general health, state of mind, and degree of stress. Women's needs for sleep are affected by their menstrual cycles as well as by pregnancy, nursing, and menopause. And everyone's need for sleep may be affected by the weather, season of the year, and amount of light he or she has been exposed to, as well as by such unusual factors as a change in altitude, time zone, or work schedule.

Thus, subjective insomniacs may be responding to a genuine lack of sleep with a faulty expression of the problem. Instead of realizing that they aren't getting as much sleep as they need, subjective insomniacs perceive the problem as "not falling asleep all night." Not getting as much sleep as one needs isn't limited to those with subjective insomnia. Many people who think they're getting enough sleep may actually be sleep-deprived. Dr. Thomas Roth of the Henry Ford

Hospital in Detroit conducted a study of the daytime sleepiness of one hundred young adults. Of those who claimed not to feel sleepy during the day, 34 percent nevertheless showed signs of excessive daytime sleepiness.

It's possible that some of the people in Roth's study were getting "enough" sleep—but perhaps their sleep wasn't sufficiently restful. Insomniacs, subjective insomniacs, and people who believe they have no sleep problems may all suffer from sleeping "inefficiently," so that even nine or ten hours of sleep leave them feeling groggy, unfocused—and envious of those who seem to breeze through life on five or six hours of sleep a night.

Many elements can affect how restful our sleep actually is. Such factors as diet and exercise can deepen sleep. The timing of our sleep—how regular our sleep schedules are, whether and for how long we nap—especially helps determine how refreshing our sleep will be. The type of bed and pillow one uses, the climate of the bedroom, the amount and type of noise that reaches the sleeper—can likewise make the difference between a restless and a restful night. And of course, both our need for sleep and our ability to sleep restfully will be affected by stress, depression, mourning, and illness.

Ironically, some people who do sleep productively and sufficiently may also be subjective insomniacs—because they themselves believe they need more sleep. As we've seen, sleep needs vary a great deal, and they tend to decrease with age. Adolescents and young adults generally need about seven and a half hours of sleep, a need that usually declines to about seven hours after age forty in men and age fifty in women. In the elderly there is interindividual variability, which precludes generalizations.

However, many adults depart from these averages, needing as few as five or as many as ten hours. Adults who only need five hours of sleep but who think they need eight may have trouble falling asleep or may wake up early in the morning—not because they're insomniacs, but because they're spending three extra hours in bed.

Some researchers have speculated that need for sleep corresponds to personality type. They point out that many well-known short sleepers were hardworking, ambitious, obsessive, extroverted, and efficient—people like Winston Churchill, Napoleon, and Voltaire. Long sleepers, on the other hand, tend to worry more and be less self-assured—but, like Albert Einstein, they're also likely to be quite creative, often passing their sleep time in vivid and adventurous dreams. Of course, there are exceptions to every rule. The moody and introverted author Fyodor Dostoevsky reportedly was a short sleeper, as was the creative inventor Thomas Edison.

In fact, no one really knows why one adult bounces through life on five or six hours while another can't function on less than nine or ten. Just as people seem to be born with particular metabolisms, so do they seem to be born with particular needs for sleep. We all know people who seem to need enormous quantities of food, even though they never gain weight, while other people genuinely seem to need only a nibble or two to satisfy their appetites. And, just as people modify their appetites and food intake based on a number of factors—diet, exercise, mental outlook, general health—so can people modify the quality of their sleep.

So whatever the nature of your particular sleep problem, take heart! You may be getting more sleep than you realize—and in any case, there are many things you can do to sleep more easily, restfully, and efficiently.

The Worst That Can Happen

The worst thing in the world is to try to sleep and not to.

—F. Scott Fitzgerald

Certainly, to an insomniac, lack of sleep seems to be its own punishment. Beyond the discomfort of the sleepless night, however, what's the worst that can happen?

The first thing to remember is that insomnia is a symptom, not a medical problem. It's a sign that something isn't working right for you, but insomnia itself isn't a disease. It may take the edge off some of the anxiety about insomnia to remember that although one or two sleepless nights can make you extremely uncomfortable, by themselves they can't really hurt you.

That's not to say that you may not feel aftereffects from sleep deprivation. Although many people don't necessarily feel tired after a single sleepless night—adrenaline helps them compensate—their judgments or reactions may be affected. They may find themselves feeling low in energy, groggy, depressed, or irritable. Some people lose their appetite. Others experience burning eyes or wobbly knees. Some people just don't feel like working when they're not well rested. Sleep loss can make people less alert, less coordinated, and somewhat less able to perform simple motor tasks. However, unless you're driving long distances or operating heavy machinery, the loss of one night of sleep probably won't seriously affect your ability to carry out your normal duties.

If you were completely deprived of sleep for several nights in a row, the consequences would be far more serious, including paranoia and hallucinations of sight, touch, or hearing. However, even after eight to eleven days of total sleep deprivation, every body part functions normally except the brain. And of course, such extreme deprivation must be deliberate—the result of a laboratory experiment or a conscious effort to keep yourself awake. Even then, after two or three days, you'll need lab personnel or friends to wake you. Next to sex and hunger, sleep is the most powerful urge we know—so even the most restless insomniac will fall asleep eventually.

What about chronic sleep deprivation—frequent sleepless nights or always getting just a few hours less sleep than you need? The effects of that pattern may come to *seem* like an illness—a feeling of listlessness, irritability, difficulty concentrating, impaired judgment. Your reaction time may be impaired. Studies have shown that a sleep-deprived person's reaction time doesn't just slow down but also becomes more erratic, at times approaching normal, at other times falling off drastically. A person's vulnerability to pain increases with exhaustion. Some people have memory problems. Others become negative, hostile, apathetic, or depressed.

More insidiously, a person might attribute these qualities to his or her emotional state, unaware that they might dissipate after more sleep. Of course, when you're depressed, stressed, or upset is also when you may have the most difficulty sleeping, creating a vicious cycle in which emotional frustrations and sleep deprivation feed on and support each other. Researchers have found that sleep loss from stress seems to affect people more intensely than the insomnia caused by overeating or travel, suggesting that your attitude about your insomnia in particular and your life in general plays a big role in determining how sleeplessness will affect you.

The good news is that the ill effects of *all* forms of insomnia—a single sleepless night, sustained sleep deprivation, chronic sleep deprivation—can be remedied relatively easily. All it takes to compensate for one lost night of sleep is an extra 25 percent of a normal night's sleep—i.e., if your normal night is eight hours long, two extra hours is all you need to erase the effects of a sleepless night.

More severe deprivation takes a bit longer to overcome, but not that much. In 1964, for example, a California high school student stayed up for eleven days straight. He functioned reasonably well even on the last day of this experiment, then went on to sleep fifteen hours straight—and felt completely recovered. Adults may need weeks.

If you've been chronically depriving yourself of sleep—periodically missing entire nights or continually getting an hour or two less than you need—you may need three to six weeks to recover the benefits of being well rested. Even then, however, you'll probably feel a great deal of improvement as soon as your sleeping habits start to change.

Ironically, anxiety about sleeping can itself cause insomnia. (Psychologists even have a word for it: *agrypniaphobia*, or fear of insomnia.) So give yourself a break. Remember that one or two sleepless nights won't kill you, and allow yourself to take the time you need to retool your sleeping patterns. An attitude of relaxed curiosity about your problem will take you a lot further than a sense of urgency.

What Are Sleep Disorders?

> I fall asleep soundly, but after an hour I wake up, as though I
> had laid my head in the wrong hole.
> I . . . have before me anew the labour of falling asleep and
> feel myself rejected by sleep.
>
> —Franz Kafka

Not all forms of insomnia are the same. In medical terminology, insomnias are grouped under a heading called DIMS — disorders of initiating or maintaining sleep. In addition to insomnias, these disorders include a number of other sleep disturbances, such as sleep apnea (in which the sleeper has difficulty breathing), periodic leg movements, and nightmares (which may cause the sleeper to awaken, perhaps with attendant difficulty in getting back to sleep).

Researchers have identified three basic ways in which people lose sleep:

〉 *Difficulty initiating sleep.* Specialists estimate that it takes a healthy sleeper from ten to fifteen minutes to fall asleep. If you fall asleep much more quickly than that, you may be sleep-deprived. If it takes you much longer than that to fall asleep, you're considered to have insomnia.

Of course, as we've seen, people's need for sleep varies, as do individuals' daily rhythms. Some people who have trouble falling asleep may simply be trying to go to bed too early, either because they're committed to getting an eight hours that they don't really need, or because they're more comfortable with a later bedtime and a later rising time than the schedule they've chosen. Some "late birds" have cured their insomnia by arranging work schedules to allow them to come into work later. Others stay up late, get up early, and find a way to take a nap during the day. (For more on naps, see Chapter 5.)

It's also striking how much our attitudes affect our ability to initiate sleep. Mark Twain, a famous insomniac, was notoriously fussy about the conditions for his rest, and so he was almost always unable to fall asleep away from home. One night when he was staying as a guest in someone's house, he tossed and turned until finally he decided that his room's stuffy air was the culprit keeping him awake. In frustration, he threw a shoe at the window and, hearing the glass smash, breathed a sigh of relief. Soon he was sleeping soundly. When he awoke the next morning, however, he found that the shoe had smashed not the window but the glass door to a book-case. Apparently, Twain's mind was a far more powerful sleep-inducer than fresh air!

) *Difficulty maintaining sleep.* This form of insomnia is what occurs when people wake frequently during the night and have trouble falling asleep again. In fact, most people wake periodically during the night, usually without being aware of it. In some sleep disorders, though, including sleep apnea and periodic leg movements, the sleeper may wake as often as four to five hundred times during the night—perhaps also without being aware of it. Nevertheless, these interruptions keep the sleeper from enjoying restful, refreshing sleep, and he or she is likely to wake up tired or groggy.

In other sleep disorders, such as nightmares, the sleeper is quite aware of being awakened from slumber. Whether the sleeper finds it easy or difficult to get back to sleep, frequent, disturbing nightmares certainly interfere with the restful quality of sleep and may also bring on a difficulty initiating sleep, as the sleeper fears the dreams that may come.

Some sleepers report waking in the middle of the night with anxiety attacks. Others are woken easily by noise—sometimes by sounds that would fail to disturb anyone else. (We know one problem sleeper who claimed to be awakened by the sound of a guest puffing on a pipe in the next room.) Still others wake for no apparent reason.

The sleep disturbance in these cases may take many forms. In some cases, it's a matter of actual minutes or hours lost from total sleep time. In other cases, the awakened sleeper has lost the deepest and most restful stage of sleep (nondreaming sleep has four stages, each deeper than the last, which alternate cyclically throughout the night; for more on sleep stages, see Chapter 2). In still other cases, the sleep disturbance is primarily psychological: the sleeper *feels* disturbed by the awakening and so feels unrested, even though, biologically speaking, he or she may have gotten adequate sleep.

) *Early awakenings.* In this form of insomnia, the sleeper has no trouble falling asleep but then wakes up far earlier than he or she would like. As with difficulties in initiating sleep, difficulties with early awakenings may be a pseudo-problem in some cases. It's quite possible that the early riser really doesn't need more than five or six hours of sleep, so his or her early mornings actually represent the gift of more time. It's also possible that the early riser does need seven, eight, or more hours but might consider an earlier bedtime rather than trying to sleep later. (If the sleeper is waking before it gets light, however, it's unlikely that this is his or her "natural" time to wake up.)

This type of sleep disorder may be particularly frustrating to ambitious, self-directed people, who'd have no trouble following a program to allow themselves to get to sleep, but who feel that an unscheduled waking time is particularly out of their control. These inadvertent early risers can't battle their problem head-on with a warm glass of milk before bedtime or a soothing nighttime routine. They don't even know whether they'll *have* a problem until they find themselves awake and unable to get back to sleep. There *are* ways to overcome unwanted early risings, of course, but the problem sleeper may have to consider more subtle changes in his or her lifestyle or outlook.

Like the other categories, unwanted early risings may also be related to anxiety and/or depression. Specialists tend to generalize that difficulty falling asleep suggests anxiety while difficulty staying asleep indicates depression, but of course, there are numerous exceptions to this rule. Certainly, people may find themselves thrust out of sleep, full of worries about an impending deadline or a foundering love affair, just as they may find that feelings of hopelessness or helplessness keep them from comfortably finding their way into sleep.

People who are depressed may also sleep more than usual. Alternately, they may experience difficulties initiating or maintaining sleep along with an increased need for sleep. Thus, a person who is depressed might go to bed at, say, 10 P.M., wake up unwillingly at 4 A.M., try for several hours to fall back to sleep without success, and finally wind up sleeping from 9 A.M. to noon. That's a total of only nine hours of sleep—yet fourteen hours have been consumed. (For more about sleep and depression, see Chapter 3.)

Insomnia may be chronic (lasting more than three weeks at a time) or transient (appearing only occasionally). Both chronic and transient insomnia may have any one of a number of causes, or be caused by a combination of factors. Here are some of the major causes of insomnias and other common sleep disorders:

❯ *Medical problems.* Although insomnia itself isn't a disease, it's often associated with other medical disorders. Respiratory problems, particularly asthma, can interfere with sleep; so can various forms of heart disease. The following chronic conditions are frequently associated with insomnia: ulcers, migraine headache, cluster headache, hyperthyroidism, hypothyroidism, arthritis, diabetes, and Parkinson's disease. Certainly, other medical conditions may be responsible for sleep disturbances as well.

❯ *Sleep apnea.* As mentioned earlier, sleep apnea is a condition that prevents normal breathing during sleep. This disorder accounts for the problems of 5 percent of insomniacs who visit sleep clinics (most people with sleep apnea sleep too easily), although it may go unnoticed and undiagnosed for years. A person with sleep apnea actually stops breathing for up to a minute at a time. The sleeper wakes up briefly, and breathing resumes again. As this may happen as often as four hundred to five hundred times in a single night, the sleeper finally awakens feeling groggy and drowsy, but often unaware of the source of the problem. Snoring is a key to sleep apnea; it's also more common in those over forty and in people with a tendency to obesity. It may be susceptible to medication or, in extreme cases, to a tracheotomy (a surgical incision in the throat that allows the sleeper to breathe direct-ly through the windpipe; the incision must be covered during the day). The treatment of choice is nasal continuous positive airway pressure (CPAP) via a mask worn during sleep.

❭ *Periodic leg movements.* Ten to twenty percent of all chronic insomnia is caused by this condition, in which the sleeper's legs jerk or move involuntarily, in bursts of twenty-five to forty seconds. Incidents of periodic leg movements may occur every few minutes over a span of several hours and may arouse the sleeper as often as four hundred times a night. Indications that you might have periodic leg move-ments include discomfort in the lower leg which requires movement for relief (restless legs syndrome), or a spouse who complains of being kicked at night. Although this disorder is not well understood, a doctor or specialist may be able to pro-vide medication that will alleviate its sleep-disturbing quali-ties.

❭ *Circadian rhythm disturbances.* All living creatures operate on cycles of various lengths. Cycles that last approxi-mately one day are known as *circadian* cycles or rhythms, from the Latin words *circa* (around) and *die* (day). Sleep pat-terns are closely linked to circadian rhythms, which have a profound and complicated effect on our ability to fall asleep and wake up at satisfying times. Changes in circadian rhythms caused by flying across time zones, changing work shifts, or simply staying up unusually late several nights in a row may cause difficulties in getting a normal night's sleep. Other factors may also affect a person's circadian rhythms, so that the sleeper can actually get a "good night's sleep"—but not during the hours that he or she might prefer (e.g., the sleeper falls asleep at 4 A.M. and sleeps till noon).

Behavioral circadian rhythm disturbances are involved in what is known as *learned insomnia*. In this type of sleep disorder, the sleeper is initially kept awake for a specific reason—possibly a series of late-night work sessions, perhaps a few nights of stress-induced insomnia. However, after the initial cause has disappeared—the workload goes back to normal, the stress dissipates—the sleeper continues to fall asleep at the new, late hour, even if he or she is also getting up regularly at an early hour.

Some circadian rhythm disturbances have obvious causes; others are harder to decipher. Either way, the solution is the same: the sleeper reconditions his or her schedule to more appropriate sleep and wake times. (For a more detailed discussion of circadian rhythms and their effects on sleep, see Chapter 5.)

〉 *Medications.* Ironically, the pills you take to make another condition better may be making your insomnia worse. Medications known to interfere with sleep include amphetamines, antidepressants, antihistamines, and birth-control pills. Sleeping pills, muscle relaxants, and other sedatives may also cause sleep problems; if you've come to rely on these medications to help you sleep (even if that's not the original reason you took them), you may find it hard to sleep without them. (For more on sleeping pills and insomnia, see Chapter 6.)

〉 *Smoking, drinking, and recreational drugs.* Anything that affects your nervous system affects your relationship to sleep—and recreational substances are no exception. Nicotine is a stimulant, like caffeine, that may affect your body's ability to relax fully into sleep. Drinking interferes with healthy sleep in numerous ways. Generally, people who drink heavily or regularly have difficulty falling asleep, and even one or two drinks at a social occasion can interfere with that night's slumber. The person who passes out or falls asleep after "one too many" may have departed from consciousness, but he or she is unlikely to experience restful sleep. Marijuana is a sedative that, if used regularly, may make it difficult for the user to fall asleep without smoking. Recreational stimulants, such as cocaine, severely interfere with the relaxation necessary for sleep. (For more on nicotine, alcohol, and drugs, see Chapter 4.)

) *Psychological factors.* As we've already said, anxiety and depression can either keep a person awake or wake a sleeper far too early. Preoccupation with emotional problems, involvement in a challenging work situation, or excitement over a wonderful new development in your professional or emotional life—getting a promotion, falling in love—can also interfere with deep, peaceful sleep. Certainly, psychological factors can interact with any of the other factors discussed here, affecting both the severity of the sleep disturbance and the sleeper's feelings about his or her insomnia.

Solving Your Sleep Problem

> Since sleep is inextricably interknit with a person's general health and way of life, it is unreasonable and illogical to expect good sleep during an inherently unhealthy life.
> Nonetheless, this is the expectation of most people.
>
> —Gay Luce and Julius Segal, *Sleep*

Most of us, when faced with a problem, try to diagnose its cause and use that information to proceed to a solution. That approach may be helpful as you try to solve your sleep problem. However, you may also find that a more playful approach, one that relies more on curiosity and less on logic, may serve you better. What's causing your sleep problem and what will cure it aren't necessarily identical. So trying out a number of different remedies, relying on your instincts of what sounds right, and keeping an open mind about what might work may be your best bet.

For example, suppose you have *learned insomnia*. Several late-night deadlines kept you up later than usual; the stress that went with the deadlines meant you didn't sleep when you did get to bed. All those extra cups of coffee, late-night cigarettes, and sugary treats probably didn't help either; neither did cutting out your usual before-dinner walk. Now, though, your work is all done, the stress has apparently passed, you've cut back to your usual level of coffee and cigarettes, you're back to one dessert a week and a regular walk after work. There seems to be no reason for your insomnia to continue—and yet you just can't get to sleep.

If this is the case, you might proceed by analyzing what caused your insomnia—late hours, stress, diet, and exercise patterns. But if every one of those factors is apparently back to normal, you might run into a dead end.

At this point, you might abandon logic and turn to intuition. How can you experiment with possible remedies for sleeplessness? Perhaps the idea of a soothing bedtime routine appeals to you. Maybe you need to increase the amount of aerobic exercise you get or adjust your diet. Possibly, you'll turn to a broader examination of your life, asking yourself whether your insomnia is a clue to deeper dissatisfactions about your work, your family, or some other aspect of your life. Or perhaps you'll avoid psychology and self-analysis altogether, deciding instead to learn to meditate. You may not need to know what's causing your insomnia in order to discover a cure. Or, alternately, the search for a cure may be a wider-ranging, deeper, and more intuitive process than you initially suspected.

Certainly, sleep problems are continuous with waking problems. Things that bother you in your waking life are very likely to plague your sleep. Diet, exercise, and attitude affect many aspects of your existence—their impact on your sleep may only be their most obvious effect. You might think of your insomnia as an invitation to explore your life more fully, to find ways of caring for your body and spirit that will ultimately be more satisfying and productive for you. In this approach, any one of a number of changes may be helpful, even if you don't know why—and any one change might lead to a myriad others.

As you read this book, you may discover that your insomnia has a deeper significance for you. Or you may find out that your sleeplessness is easily addressed with a simple change or two—cutting out that after-dinner coffee, adding a daily ten-minute walk, drinking a glass of milk before bedtime. You may find ways of sleeping more productively and restfully. You might even decide that you don't have insomnia after all—you just don't need as much sleep as you thought.

Whatever you finally decide, remember that your sleep—or the lack of it—is an integral part of your life as a whole. Physical changes become emotional changes, and vice versa. Insomnia is a striking example of how mind and body, emotion and thought, physical health and mental attitude, are profoundly interrelated. This book will give you the resources to explore many different areas of mind, body, and spirit. The rest is up to you.

What's in This Book

This book will address many aspects of sleeplessness and "sleep cures." In Chapter 2, you can find out more about the biology of sleep and the nature of dreaming. You'll also find help preparing a sleep journal and a sleep history, which you can use either to diagnose your problem yourself or to work with a doctor or sleep specialist. Finally, you'll learn some ways to cut down on your amount of time in bed, so that you can actually spend less time, as well as sleep more easily.

Chapter 3 examines the psychological components of insomnia—how it relates to stress and depression, how it may be your way of giving yourself a hidden message. The chapter also offers suggestions for finding and working with a therapist or counselor, describing the various types of therapies that are available.

Chapter 4 explores diet. You'll find out which foods help keep you awake and which will ease your path to sleep. You'll also learn how cigarettes, alcohol, recreational drugs, and many common medications affect your ability to sleep.

In Chapter 5, you'll learn more about circadian rhythms, those daily cycles that play such an important role in our ability to sleep and wake when we choose. You'll find out how naps can affect your daytime alertness as well as your nighttime sleep. And you'll learn to tune in to your own unique rhythms.

Chapter 6 looks at both medical and natural remedies for insomnia. After reading the latest information on over-the-counter and prescription sleep aids, you'll go on to learn about other ways of coping with stress. Many people have successfully addressed insomnia with exercise, meditation, and biofeedback. In this chapter, you'll learn more about these and other techniques. The chapter will also examine alternative medical practices—homeopathy, chiropractic, the Chinese tradition of acupuncture and herbal medicine, and the Ayurvedic medical tradition of India.

Finally, in Chapter 7, you'll find help in creating a good sleep setting—a comfortable bed, a relaxing bedroom, a soothing environment. You'll also find a number of helpful suggestions for courting sleep, including hints for establishing a bedtime routine.

Arriving at peaceful, refreshing sleep may happen very quickly for you. Or it may take you some time to find your way to the sleep patterns you'd prefer. Either way, the journey can be rewarding, offering you a chance to learn more about yourself and to make your entire life—waking and sleeping—more satisfying. This book can be your resource, but in the end, you are the final authority on what will work for you. Noted sleep expert Dr. Wilse Webb once called sleep "the gentle tyrant." But with enough time and patience, you can turn the tyrant into a friend.

Chapter 2

How Tired Are You?

Despite fifty years of research, all we can conclude about the function of sleep is that it overcomes sleepiness, and the only reliable finding from sleep deprivation experiments is that sleep loss makes us sleepy.

—Dr. James Horne, *Why We Sleep*

We spend almost one-third of our lives sleeping. Yet no one knows why. True, sleep researchers have developed a few theories, but so far sleep remains one of life's great mysteries.

Although scientists know little about why we sleep, they do know quite a bit about *how* sleep proceeds. That's fortunate, because this knowledge can help each of us better understand what does and doesn't work for us when it comes to our own sleep patterns.

Before going on to find out more about scientists' and doctors' views of sleep, however, you might want to pause and remember how important *you* are in the process of diagnosing and curing your sleep problems. You have an important part to play in any treatment you receive, but your role is particularly important with a disorder like insomnia, which can be affected by so many tangible and intangible factors. As you continue to read about the biology of sleep, you might want to keep the following key points in mind:

) No one knows exactly how much sleep *you* need. That's something only you can determine, through trial and error.

) The quality of your sleep is alterable. Diet, exercise, and life changes can all affect your sleep.

) Your ideas about yourself and how much sleep you need are significant, both in determining how much sleep you need, and in enabling you to find sleeping patterns that are comfortable for you.

Therefore, after going through the latest scientific theories about sleep, this chapter concludes with a section designed to help you explore your own sleep patterns—a detailed questionnaire to help you explore your relationship to sleep, along with suggestions for keeping a sleep journal and writing a sleep history. You can use these tools either on your own or with a doctor, other health professional, or therapist. (For more on working with a doctor, see Chapter 3.)

Why Sleep?

The fact is, from a strictly neurological and physiological viewpoint, there is no objective proof that any restorative or recuperative processes get under way [during sleep]. And yet we all know, subjectively, that sleep makes us feel better— that we feel refreshed by a good night's sleep and feel miserable when we are sleepless.

—Dr. Peter Hauri, director, Sleep Center, Mayo Clinic

Scientists have advanced many theories about our need for sleep. Some are conflicting, others may peacefully coexist. It's also true that processes that occur *during* sleep may not be the reason *for* sleep. For example, we rest during sleep—but if we rest without sleeping, we feel somewhat deprived. Although rest occurs during sleep, that alone doesn't account for why we sleep.

Certainly, the question of why we sleep is an intriguing one when you consider how vulnerable we are during these six to ten hours. To quote University of Chicago sleep-researcher Allan Rechtschaffen, "If sleep does not serve an absolutely vital function, then it is the biggest mistake the evolutionary process ever made."

Other animals, even other mammals, remain far closer to wakefulness during sleep than humans do, suggesting that for them, at least, the evolutionary process recognized and responded to the state's potential danger. Giraffes, for example, sleep only for three to seventy-five minutes at a time, for a total of two hours of sleep out of twenty-four. But then, the giraffe needs fifteen seconds just to stand up, so you can imagine how vulnerable it is in sleep. Nevertheless, even the giraffe lies down three to eight times a night, so the need for sleep—as opposed to relaxed wakefulness—must be very great indeed.

Dolphins, porpoises, and seals must sleep while they're afloat. Sleep exposes them both to the risk of drowning and to the danger of being eaten by their enemies. The blind Indus dolphin copes by sleeping only ninety seconds at a time, for a total of seven hours out of twenty-four. Other sea mammals have evolved an ingenious three-hour sleep-wake cycle: one hour with the right hemisphere of the brain asleep while the left remains awake, one hour when the left sleeps and the right stays awake, and one hour where both are asleep. The complexity of this system attests both to the risks involved in sleep—and to the overwhelming need for it.

One theory holds that sleep is a kind of forced time out. Related theories suggest that sleep was a primitive mechanism developed when food was perpetually scarce: the reduced amount of physical exertion resulting from sleep helped reduce our need for food.

However, scientists have been unable to determine why sleep, rather than simply relaxation, is necessary to overcome muscular fatigue. According to prominent Stanford sleep-researcher Dr. William C. Dement, "While it is true that muscular fatigue will be ameliorated while the body is 'at rest' during the night, it seems clear that reversal of fatigue is not the specific function of sleep or the sole reason for its existence." Since people who are bedridden twenty-four hours a day seem to need just as much sleep as active people, the notion that sleep is primarily a resting time seems unsatisfying.

After all, although small-brained mammals like mice and rabbits don't seem able to relax or stop moving unless they're asleep, large-brained mammals like humans are perfectly capable of resting while awake. Why, then, isn't resting without sleep enough to make us alert?

Another possibility is that sleep offers a respite from emotional tension. If we imagine the stresses undergone by prehistoric humans, their constant need to seek food and defend from danger, the idea that sleep offers a "time out" seems logical in a way. Yet many people find dreams an emotional experience, and certainly they may be a time when our emotions tell us we're in danger, even though dream dangers are imaginary.

A related idea is that sleep is an opportunity to purge psychic stress, via the process of dreaming. Founder of psychoanalysis Sigmund Freud called dreams "the royal road to the unconscious," and started an entire psychoanalytic tradition in which dreams were seen as the psyche's attempt to resolve conflicts that it could not face consciously during the day.

Alternately, Nobel Prize–winner Francis Crick suggests that sleep is a time for the brain to "dump" all of its excess mental and emotional baggage through dreams—that dreams are, in effect, the equivalent of erasing useless or outmoded files from a computer, leaving more space free for the next day's work. Far from being clues to the deepest mysteries of our soul, dreams for Crick are the garbage we must toss out, the mental and emotional clutter we must clear away. Whereas Freud theorized that we often forget dreams because their content is too emotionally charged, Crick suggests that in fact, dreams are meant to be forgotten. (For more about dreaming, see below.)

It seems clear that sleep plays some kind of role in restoring the body and/or the brain, but the exact nature of this role is still unclear to us. Some scientists point to the increased rate of elimination of metabolic waste products during sleep. Others remind us that the ongoing replacement of cells in the body intensifies during sleep. However, both elimination of waste and replacement of cells also take place during the day, so it isn't clear whether sleep is crucial to these processes.

Certainly, sleep helps the mind work better. Sleep-deprivation experiments show that subjects quickly lose mental abilities when they're operating on insufficient sleep, while one study of schoolchildren found that students who were two to three years behind their peers quickly caught up when they were encouraged to get more sleep.

It's possible that sleep's function is to allow some of the brain to rest. While our bodies can relax during wakefulness, our minds cannot. As long as we're conscious, our sensory apparatus is continually registering information, which the brain processes. When we're asleep, we're by definition *not* conscious of the world around us, allowing brain activity to subside.

Of course, the brain is quite active during dreams. In fact, you might say we lose consciousness of the world around us in order to focus exclusively on the world within us. During the dreamless portions of sleep, however, which make up about three-quarters of our night's rest, certain types of brain functions do decrease.

The restorative function of sleep may also relate to hormonal and/or endocrine activity. We know that certain hormonal activity peaks during sleep, particularly that of the human growth hormone (HGH), which helps to synthesize protein, promote growth, and repair damaged tissue. If you've noticed that a cut seems to have healed during sleep, human growth hormone helped the new tissue to grow.

By the same token, the hormone parathormone, regulating the level of calcium in the blood, peaks during the final hours of sleep. Prolactin, which helps nursing mothers produce milk, peaks at about the same time. However, the coincidence of hormonal activity and sleep doesn't mean that sleep is necessary for hormonal activity.

Recent research has taken off in a new direction, relating sleep to the immune system. University of Toronto psychiatrist Harvey Moldofsky found that the blood's level of

T lymphocytes—the cells that destroy abnormal cells—are far lower during sleep than during wakefulness. Moldofsky speculates that the T cells have left the blood to go out into the body, attacking abnormal cells while we sleep.

Another of Moldofsky's findings is the discovery that our blood's level of B cells, which form antibodies, is considerably higher during sleep. Perhaps the body is arming itself with antibodies at night so that it can prevent the invasion of "foreign" germs the next day.

Further evidence for this line of thinking comes from studies of hospital patients which reveal that patients recuperate much faster when allowed to sleep as much as they want. In one study, older people found relief from chronic fatigue and depression when they were allowed to sleep longer. Another study found that sleep helped relieve the symptoms of women who were tired, run-down, and nervous.

It seems that we need more sleep when we feel sick, and we're more likely to *get* sick when we haven't been getting enough sleep. Happily, Moldofsky has also discovered that the immune system is resilient. Even after subjects have been deprived of sleep for forty hours straight, one good night's sleep was all they needed for their immune systems to return to full strength.

Sleep in Other Cultures

Sleep is the most moronic fraternity in the world, with the heaviest dues and the crudest rituals.

—Vladimir Nabokov

Our notion of the eight-hour night is so ingrained that we've come to think of it as a biological necessity. All we need to do to dispel that notion, however, is to look at the wide range of sleep patterns existing in other cultures.

Before the industrial revolution and the tyranny of the clock—that is, for the major part of human history—most cultures were primarily agricultural. People tended to go to sleep when it became dark and rise when the sun came up. Thus, in winter, people slept longer, while in summer they seemed to get along on less sleep. In some parts of the world today, people still sleep up to twelve hours a night in winter while sleeping only about six hours in summer. Scandinavian countries, for example, tend to operate by nature's clock rather than by a more regularized year-round system.

The Masai, an African people, sleep far less than most people in the United States: the men sleep about three to four hours a night, the women somewhat longer. Likewise, the Temiar of Malaysia sleep about six hours a night. Of course, genetics, diet, exercise, and lifestyle play a role in the sleep patterns that work for various peoples, but it's heartening to know that the biology of sleep is far more elastic than we might think. Even in the United States, two people in ten sleep less than six hours a night, according to the National Center for Health Statistics.

The Different Stages of Sleep

When you start to ask the question, "What is the function of sleep?" it's the same as asking "What is the function of wakefulness?" I don't know the function of being awake any more than I know the function of being asleep.

—Dr. Anthony Kales

Despite the huge variations in styles and amounts of sleep, there are some aspects of sleep that all humans share. Since the 1930s, we have had at our disposal noninvasive techniques for measuring electrical activity in the brain, allowing people to be studied while they were actually asleep. In 1952, University of Chicago sleep-researcher Nathaniel Kleitman discovered that although sleepers tended to have slow, rolling eye movements beneath their lids as they fell asleep, during some portions of their sleep their eyes darted rapidly in a highly coordinated way, moving more quickly and sharply than they could while the subject was awake. Kleitman dubbed the phenomenon *rapid eye movement*, a phase of sleep that was later related to dreaming.

Using an electroencephalogram (EEG)—a device that measures electrical activity in the brain, or *brain waves*—researchers eventually realized that the REM stage of sleep is as different from non-REM (NREM) sleep as sleep is from waking. This groundbreaking discovery implied that rather than being a time of shutdown, sleep was actually quite an active state. Not only were dreams produced by one center of the brain during the REM phase, but the rapid eye movements themselves were produced by quite a different part of the brain. Penile erections are also common in men during this phase of sleep, and they appear to be caused by yet another part of the brain. Whatever restorative function sleep serves, it does not accomplish this function through lack of activity!

Later research determined that NREM sleep is further divided into four stages, representing a progression into deeper stages. The pattern and continuity of sleep stages during the night determine how restful and refreshing our sleep is—and may offer valuable clues to those of us trying to improve the quality of our sleep.

The initial stage of sleep—the time of falling asleep—is known as the *threshold*. Although the term *falling asleep* makes the process sound gradual and progressive, it occurs in seconds. In one experiment, people who were trying to fall asleep with their eyes open were shown bright flashes of light ever second or so. They were instructed to press a switch whenever they saw a flash. Each subject continued to press the switch regularly—until suddenly, responses just stopped. When you switch over into sleep, your awareness of the outside world vanishes in seconds.

Relaxation just prior to sleep is characterized by a steady, even alpha rhythm (*alpha* signifies a pattern of brain-wave activity, representing short, relatively frequent waves). Gradually, muscular tension decreases and bodily functions slow down. The sleeper's mind wanders, and his or her awareness grows dull.

Then the sleeper enters the so-called Stage 1 of non-REM sleep. Breathing becomes slow and even, the heartbeat becomes regular, blood pressure falls, brain temperature decreases, the blood flow to the brain is reduced, and there is little body movement. Generally, this description of bodily functions characterizes all non-REM sleep.

Stage 1 sleep might be called a kind of twilight time. It's initial appearance lasts up to ten minutes in most sleepers. Brain waves become smaller, slower, somewhat irregular. This portion of sleep is characterized by drifting thoughts and dreams that move from the real to the fantastic, along with a kind of floating feeling. At this point, the sleeper is still easily awakened and might even deny having slept. Stage 1 sleep is the period we might call "drifting off."

From Stage 1, the sleeper will gradually descend deeper into sleep, becoming more and more detached from the outside world and progressively more difficult to awaken. Stage 2, an intermediate stage of sleep, initially lasts about twenty minutes. It is characterized by larger brain waves and occasional quick bursts of activity. The sleeper may be vaguely conscious of some thoughtlike fragments floating through the brain but will not see anything even if the eyes are opened. Bodily functions continue to slow down, so that blood pressure, metabolism, secretions, and cardiac activity are all decreased. (You can see how the body's need to digest a large meal would militate against its need to slow down in this way. For more on sleep and digestion, see Chapter 4.)

Nevertheless, a sleeper in Stage 2 is still easily awakened by sounds. In Stage 3, by contrast, the sleeper is far more difficult to awaken. It takes a louder noise or an active attempt to wake him or her. Stage 3 brain waves are slow—coming at the rate of one per second—and quite large—five times the size of waves in Stage 2. In fact, Stage 3 brain waves are known as delta waves. Stage 3 is the beginning of deep sleep, occurring about thirty to forty five minutes after you first fall asleep.

The deepest sleep occurs in Stage 4. The delta brain waves are quite large, making a slow, jagged pattern on the EEG. At this point, the sleeper experiences virtual oblivion. If the sleeper is a sleepwalker or a bed wetter, those activities will begin in this phase. Children who get night terrors—awakening with a nonspecific feeling of fear, as opposed to waking from a nightmare—will get them during this phase of sleep. Bodily functions, however, are continuing to decline to the deepest possible state of physical rest.

Some theorists have lumped Stages 3 and 4 together into one phase called "deep sleep" or "slow wave sleep." Together, the two stages may last only a few minutes or up to an hour. (In children, this phase lasts much longer, however.)

Although the sleeper may repeat the cycle of NREM sleep another two times during the night, this first period of deep sleep is the deepest. The sleeper awakened from deep sleep will probably be groggy, confused, or disoriented. He or she may experience "sleep inertia" or "sleep drunkenness," seeming unable to function normally for quite some time.

You may have had the experience of waking a child during this phase of sleep. You can steer a child in deep sleep into the bathroom, for example, but the child clearly is not aware of anything that is going on.

Once again, the special nature of deep sleep raises questions about sleep's functions in our lives. It would seem quite dangerous for humans and other mammals to experience a biological state of unconsciousness from which it is quite difficult to be aroused—one might think that it would better serve the organism to be ever ready to wake and flee from danger. Yet the low arousability of sleepers in deep sleep insures that sleep will continue, so it must serve some very important function.

After the first phase of deep sleep ends, the sleeper returns to Stage 2 and then enters the REM state. As we've seen, the rapid eye movements aren't actually a response to dreams. About 85 percent of the REM phase is passed in dreaming.

Brain waves during the REM state are small and irregular, with big bursts of eye activity. In many ways, brainwave activity at this time resembles waking more than it does sleeping.

As opposed to the progressive relaxation of the four NREM phases, the body's activity perks up considerably during the REM phase. Blood pressure becomes variable but may increase drastically. Pulse rates increase in an irregular way as well, and the sleeper with cardiac problems faces his or her greatest risk of heart attack at this time. Breathing becomes irregular and oxygen consumption increases.

The chin is slack during REM sleep, but the face as well as the toes and fingers may twitch. A man experiences penile erections during this phase, while a woman experiences clitoral engorgement. However, sleepers' large muscles are literally paralyzed, so that they cannot move their torsos, arms, or legs. That seems to be our bodies' way of keeping us from taking physical action in response to our dreams, which, to our sleeping minds, often have all the reality of our waking state.

Normally, the body attempts to keep its own temperature at a steady 98.6 degrees Fahrenheit, but this effort is apparently abandoned during the REM phase. Shivering and sweating—bodily attempts to restore its preferred temperature—cease at this time, and the body's temperature drifts gradually toward the temperature of its environment.

After the first REM period, which is brief, you may wake up briefly. This is not necessarily indicative of bad sleep, and a sleeper who wakes at this time may not remember it the next day. A poor sleeper, on the other hand, may wake up at this point and have difficulty getting back to sleep.

In either case, the sleeper returns to Stage 1 sleep and begins the entire cycle over again. Sleepers alternate between REM and NREM sleep four to six times a night, with each cycle lasting an average of 90 minutes, with an average range of 70 to 110 minutes.

Although deep sleep dominates the first two sleep cycles, it occurs less frequently as the night wears on. That is, after your first two sleep cycles, you probably won't get any more deep sleep. On the other hand, you'll get a lot more REM time.

For reasons we don't yet understand, the dreams you remember after being awakened out of REM sleep have a far different quality from those you remember after waking up from NREM sleep. Post-REM dreams are more vivid, visual, continuous, and detailed. They seem to have a more intense emotional content, occasionally featuring bizarre or absurd stories, and are more likely to be frightening than post-NREM dreams.

Although you spend about 10 percent of your life dreaming, dreams are elusive. Most people don't remember most of their dreams, although laboratory experiments have shown that if a sleeper is wakened during the REM phase, he or she will remember the dream. Generally, though, dreams dissipate within seconds of awakening unless the dreamer makes a special effort at recall.

A detailed exploration of dream theories is beyond the scope of this book. However, you might consider enlisting your dreams to help you understand more about your sleep— or about any other issues in your life. Keep a notebook by your bed. Ask yourself as soon as you awaken what you dreamt, and tell yourself the story of your dream in your mind. Putting your dream into words will help you remember it. Then reach for your notebook and write down what you remember. You may find that other images come to mind as you write, as well as thoughts, feelings, and possible interpretations.

Even if an immediate interpretation suggests itself, you might want to allow yourself to continue to ruminate about your dream, particularly if it was joyous, disturbing, or emotionally powerful in some other way. Like works of art, dreams have multiple, often contradictory meanings. According to theories developed by psychoanalyst Carl Gustav Jung, all of the elements in your dream represent aspects of yourself (in addition to also representing other things), so other parts of your personality may be giving valuable assistance or advice to the "you-character" in the dream, even if it doesn't seem that way at first.

If you're concerned about a particular problem, you might "ask for" a dream about it as you drift off to sleep. Put your request into simple, positive language: "I want a dream to help me with my marriage." "I want a dream about my job." "I want a dream to teach me about my sleep." Don't think about the problem itself—that will probably keep you awake. Focus instead on the possibility that the answers are within you, and that your own dream will help you discover them.

Then, when you awake in the morning (or, possibly, in the middle of the night), be ready to ask yourself what you dreamt. If at first you concentrate on remembering the dream, rather than understanding it, you'll probably remember more. If you wake up in the middle of the night with the dream, write it down, but then allow yourself to wait until morning to think about it further. Remind yourself that you can think later and tell yourself, "Now is the time for sleeping."

Mysterious though they are, dreams seem to be crucial to our well-being. If a person is deprived of REM, he or she will try to make up for it somehow, often entering "REM rebound," in which the REM phase of sleep occurs far more often and far sooner than it normally does. Sleeping pills and other medications suppress both deep sleep and the REM phase of sleep, which is one reason why they may cause people to feel even more sleepy the next day.

Experiments have shown that if sleepers are awakened as soon as REM starts, they enter REM sleep more rapidly the next time, and their REM is more intense. If the deprivation continues, they go into REM as soon as they fall asleep. It becomes impossible to deprive them of REM sleep without keeping them awake all the time. Although it usually takes about ninety minutes for REM sleep to begin, as we've seen, REM-deprived people go into REM more quickly than that in shorter naps.

However, there's no evidence that deprivation of REM causes any kind of serious or long-lasting psychological problems. True, a person deprived of sleep for several days will experience paranoia, hallucinations, and other symptoms that mimic those of psychiatric disorders, but these symptoms disappear as soon as the person has been allowed to sleep again. And many studies have shown that depressed people actually benefit from the suppression of REM sleep caused by antidepressants or by limiting their sleep time to fewer hours. By the same token, no one has yet discovered any ill effects from the long-term use of antidepressants. It seems that dreaming, like sleep, remains a mystery.

What is clear, though, is that poor sleepers tend to spend less time in deep sleep, particularly Stage 4, as well as less time in REM. Poor sleepers also seem to experience wakefulness between cycles more often and for longer periods than more efficient sleepers. If you're feeling that your sleep isn't as restful and refreshing as you'd like, you might consider looking at ways to extend the time you spend in deep sleep and REM.

What daytime activities militate against these stages of sleep? Alcohol and caffeine tend to decrease a sleeper's time in deep sleep—that's why people often feel tired after a night of drinking, even if they sleep late the next day, and why people who give up caffeine report getting by with more energy on less time in bed. Nicotine, processed sugar and sweeteners, and recreational drugs also interfere with these stages of sleep, as do many prescription medications. (For more on diet and sleep, see Chapter 4.) And, again while sleeping pills help the sleeper into unconsciousness, they don't promote restful sleep; in fact, they reduce the amount of time spent in deep sleep and REM. (For more about sleeping pills, see Chapter 6.)

It's also good to know that in childhood, total sleep and REM sleep decrease, and that in adulthood deep sleep decreases. Newborns apparently spend 50 percent of their sleep time in the REM phase (prematurely born children spend even more time—up to 80 percent for an infant born at thirty weeks of gestation). During early childhood, the amount of time spent in REM sleep approaches adult levels, and it remains constant for the rest of life.

Likewise, newborn infants need sixteen hours of sleep for every twenty-four-hour day, but by age six, children need only nine hours of sleep. By age twelve, they're down to eight hours of sleep, a total that drops to an average of seven and a half by adulthood.

And by the same token, young adults spend some 25 percent of their sleep time in deep sleep, but adults aged fifty to sixty spend 10 percent or less of their sleep time sleeping deeply. Many older adults worry that they've developed insomnia, when they're only responding to a typical pattern of aging.

Sleep Journals and Sleep Histories

He who does not understand the past is condemned to repeat it.

—Santayana

Keeping a sleep journal can help you better understand your sleep patterns. In a sleep journal, you record your sleep patterns every day for at least two weeks. Besides noting how you experienced sleeping, waking, and dreaming, you write information about diet, exercise, work and family life, emotional reactions, and any other factors that are important in your life during that period. This helps you notice how events in your waking life and disturbances in your sleep may be related, as well as what things are working for you in both waking and sleep. You can use this information by yourself or you might decide to share it with a doctor or sleep specialist. Either way, you may make some useful discoveries.

Likewise, writing a sleep history can help illuminate your relationship to sleep. Whereas a sleep journal proceeds day by day, so that you only notice the patterns afterward, looking back, writing a sleep history invites you to take a long look at your entire relationship to sleep. It, too, can be extremely useful—to you alone, to your partnership with a medical doctor or health practitioner, or in your work with a counselor or therapist.

People approach sleep journals and sleep histories in different ways. You might wish to write a sleep history first, then keep a journal, then write a second sleep history or an addition based on the new insights you've gotten from your journal. You may wish to write a history slowly, over the time you're keeping your journal, or quickly, either before or after your journal work begins. You may find that the idea of either a history or a journal appeals to you, but not both. These are your tools for exploring your relationship to sleep—give them a chance, but use them as your intuition guides you.

You'll find more specific suggestions for a journal and a history below, but first, to help get you started, you might want to complete the following questionnaire. Certain patterns or insights may emerge even as you answer the questions. You might keep a notebook by your side as you read through the quiz, so you can jot down any thoughts that come to mind.

Some people also find that thinking about their sleep—particularly when they're having insomnia or other sleep troubles—is upsetting, exciting, or emotionally charged in some other way. You might jot down feelings, questions, fears, and wishes as they arise, using your writings as a jumping-off point for further exploration.

Finally, you might want to share all or part of this questionnaire with your sleeping partner. You may be surprised to find that he or she has quite a different sense of your sleep habits than you do. What you learn may be illuminating. You might even want to take the quiz together, recording your answers side by side on two columns of the same page.

WHAT I KNOW ABOUT MY SLEEP

1. I sleep soundly:
   a. almost every night
   b. most nights
   c. less often than I'd like
   d. never

2. I wake up during the night:
   a. almost every night
   b. most nights
   c. more often than I'd like
   d. never

3. I wake up earlier than I'd like:
   a. almost every morning
   b. most mornings
   c. more often than I'd like
   d. never

4. During the work week, I usually get _____ hours of sleep. During the work week, I usually get between _____ and _____ hours of sleep.

5. On the weekend (or my equivalent time off), I usually get _____ hours of sleep. On the weekend (or equivalent), I usually get between _____ and _____ hours of sleep.

6. In the past few years, the amount of sleep I get during the work week has changed:
   a. not at all

 b. somewhat
 c. drastically

Explain: _____

_____

_____

7. In the past few years, the amount of sleep I get during the weekend (or equivalent) has changed:
 a. not at all
 b. somewhat
 c. drastically

Explain: _____

_____

_____

8. During the work week, I usually go to bed:
 a. before 10 P.M.
 b. between 10 P.M. and 12 A.M.
 c. between 12 A.M. and 2 A.M.
 d. after 2 A.M.

9. On the weekend (or equivalent), I usually go to bed:
 a. before 10 P.M.
 b. between 10 P.M. and 12 A.M.
 c. between 12 A.M. and 2 A.M.
 d. after 2 A.M.

10. During the work week, I usually get up:
 a. before 6 A.M.
 b. between 6 A.M. and 8 A.M.

c. between 8 A.M. and 10 A.M.
d. after 10 A.M.

11. On the weekend (or equivalent), I usually get up:
   a. before 6 A.M.
   b. between 6 A.M. and 8 A.M.
   c. between 8 A.M. and 10 A.M.
   d. after 10 A.M.

12. Generally, I'd say my sleep schedule is:
   a. very regular
   b. somewhat regular
   c. not at all regular

13. When I wake up for the last time in the morning, I usually feel:
   a. completely wide awake and alert
   b. awake but not yet alert
   c. groggy
   d. sleepy and unwilling to wake up

14. Describe any changes in your patterns of waking up and/ or your feelings about it. If you have markedly different feelings about waking up during the work week or on weekends (or equivalent), describe and explain them. _____
_____
_____
_____
_____

15. When I get into bed at night, I fall asleep:

    a. in less than 15 minutes
    b. in 15 to 30 minutes
    c. in 30 to 45 minutes
    d. in 45 to 60 minutes
    e. after more than an hour

16. The best description for how I feel about the *amount* of sleep I get is:
    a. very satisfied
    b. somewhat satisfied
    c. somewhat dissatisfied
    d. not at all satisfied

17. If I could make one wish about my sleep, it would be ___

_____

_____

because _____

_____

18. The last time I fell asleep easily was _____

My thoughts about that are _____

_____

19. The last time I slept soundly all through the night was ___

My thoughts about that are _____

_____

20. The last time I woke up feeling rested and refreshed was
_____

My thoughts about that are _____
_____
_____

21. The thing I believe most interferes with my sleep is
_____

Other factors that I think are interfering with my sleep are
_____

How I feel about that is _____
_____
_____

22. My sleeping patterns have/have not changed in the following ways: _____
_____
_____

I believe the reasons for this are _____
_____
_____

23. I use the following substances:
____ coffee   _____
                               how much / how often / when

____ alcohol   _____
                               how much / how often / when

____ cigarettes   _____
                               how much / how often / when

___ over-the-counter
    sleeping pills
                    _____
                    how much / how often / when

___ prescription
    sleeping pills
                    _____
                    how much / how often / when

___ over-the counter
    medications
                    _____
                    how much / how often / when

___ prescription
    medications
                    _____
                    how much / how often / when

How I feel about my use of these substances is _____

_____

_____

24. My medical problems include the following:

_____

_____

I believe they affect my sleep in the following ways:

_____

_____

25. When I can't sleep at night, what I usually do is _____

_____

How I usually feel is _____

_____

_____

26. What I do during the day to make sure I sleep well at night is _____

27. I take daytime naps:
  a. almost every day
  b. almost every workday
  c. almost every weekend (or equivalent) day
  d. sometimes
  e. occasionally
  f. almost never

28. My naps usually last ____ minutes.

29. My napping patterns and desires have/have not changed in the following ways: _____
_____
_____

because _____
_____
_____
_____
_____

30. I snore:
  a. often
  b. sometimes
  c. rarely
  d. never
(You might ask your sleeping partner to confirm this. If you don't agree, note both opinions.)

31. My sleeping partner complains of being kicked at night:
  a. often
  b. sometimes

c. rarely

d. never

32. The following factors affect how well I sleep (check all that apply):

___ sleeping alone

___ sleeping with a partner

___ having sex before sleep

___ quarreling before sleep

The relationship issues that most affect my sleep are _____

_____

How I feel about that is _____

_____

33. My bedroom is:

dark/not dark

noisy/quiet

hot/cold/comfortable

humid/stuffy/dry/comfortable

34. My bed is: too hard/too soft/just right

My pillow is: too hard/too soft/just right

My bedcovers are: too heavy/too short/too binding/just right

35. How I feel about my bedroom and my sleeping conditions is _____

_____

36. I bring work home to do at night:

a. always

b. often

c. sometimes

d. rarely

e. never

How I feel about this is _____

_____

37. What I usually do the last hour before I sleep before a workday is _____

_____

38. What I usually do the last hour before I sleep before a weekend (or equivalent day off) is _____

_____

39. Now that I've completed this questionnaire, the thing I'm most struck by is _____

_____

_____

_____

$\mathcal{M}$Y SLEEP HISTORY

What I notice about how sleep varies between my work week and my time off is:

_____

_____

_____

_____

_____

_____

What I notice about how diet, exercise, and other physical factors affect my sleep is:

_____

_____

_____

_____

What I notice about how my level of stress, work and family life, relationship to my sleeping partner(s), and other emotional issues affect my sleep is:

_____

_____

_____

_____

What I notice about how holidays, family reunions, and other major events affect my sleep is:

_____

_____

_____

_____

Here's what I remember about sleep from when I was a child:

_____

_____

_____

_____

. . . when I was a teenager:

_____

_____

_____

. . . when I first left home:

_____

_____

_____

_____

. . . when I had my first "real" job:

_____

_____

_____

. . . from other important phases of my life:

_____

_____

_____

Life changes that produce stress often create difficulties in sleeping. Here's a description of the life changes I've experienced (see list below), when they occurred, and how I believe they affected my sleep:

_____

_____

_____

_____

_____

_____

_____

_____

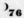

Life Changes That Can Affect Sleep

The following list was compiled by University of Washington psychiatrist T. H. Holmes, who listed changes in the order of most stressful to least stressful. Note that even positive life changes can create stress—and affect sleep.

Death of spouse
Divorce
Marital separation
Jail term
Death of close family member
Personal injury or illness
Marriage
Dismissal at work
Reconciliation with mate
Retirement
Changed health in family member
Pregnancy
Sexual difficulties
New family member
Business readjustment
Changed financial status
Death of a close friend
New type of work
Increased arguments with mate
New mortgage or loan
Foreclosure of mortgage or loan
Changed responsibilities at work
Child leaving home
In-law troubles

Outstanding personal achievement
Mate starting a new job, losing a job, or retiring
Changed living conditions
Changes in personal habits
Trouble with boss
Changed work hours or conditions
New residence
New school
Changed recreational patterns
New church activities
New social activities
A change in how often the family socializes
   or convenes
Changed eating habits
Vacation
Christmas or other major holiday
Minor violation of the law

My Sleep Journal

Day   Date   Not asleep _____ Asleep _____
6 7 8 9 10 11 12 1 2 3 4 5 6 7 8 9 10 11 12 1 2 3 4 5

Total hours of sleep _____
      Night sleep _____ Daytime sleep _____
Total hours in bed, intending to sleep _____

Yesterday's daytime activities:

_____

How I felt during the day:

_____

Yesterday's evening activities:

_____

How I felt during the evening:

_____

How I spent the last hour yesterday before I went to bed intending to sleep:

_____

How I felt about that hour:

_____

I   did/did not use an alarm clock to wake up this morning.
I   did/did not take sleeping pills last night.
If so, what I took was _____

How I felt upon waking was _____

Yesterday, for breakfast, I ate:

_____

For lunch, I ate:

_____

For dinner, I ate:

_____

Yesterday, I also consumed (including all snacks, cigarettes, alcoholic beverages, prescription drugs, and recreational drugs):

_____

_____

_____

Comments: _____

_____

_____

_____

_____

_____

_____

_____

_____

_____

Rating myself on the following scale, here's how I felt yesterday:

First thing in the morning _____

Two hours after waking _____

At lunchtime _____

Two hours after lunch _____

At dinnertime _____

Two hours after dinner _____

At bedtime _____

Scale

1 very tired

2 somewhat tired

3 all right

4 alert, energetic

5 very alert and
  energetic

Comments: _____
_____
_____
_____
_____
_____
_____
_____
_____
_____
_____
_____
_____
_____
_____
_____
_____

Deciding to Work with a Doctor

> The insomniac patient should be made to understand that he
> or she must take charge of his own life. Don't take your body
> to the doctor as if he were a repair shop.
>
> —Dr. Quentin Regestein

When is it time to get a doctor's help in solving your
sleep problems? And if you do decide to work with a doctor,
what should you expect from and bring to the relationship?

Deciding when to work with a doctor must be an individual decision, of course. A lot will depend on the relationship you have with your physician. Is he or she willing to work with you on a number of nondrug treatments, such as exercise, meditation, and relaxation exercises? Is your physician skilled in nutrition and aware of how different foods affect your ability to sleep? Is your doctor interested in issues of "wellness"? Does he or she tend to prescribe medication routinely, or only as a last resort? Will he or she refer you to a sleep specialist, if unable to fully solve your problems?

It's best if you can solve your sleep problems without using medication. Although many doctors prescribe sleeping pills and antianxiety drugs routinely, sleep specialists agree that medication is useful for only the most temporary of sleep problems. Basically, taking sleep medication can help you sleep for three days to a week; after that, the pills tend to become ineffective, besides posing a risk of several severe side effects. (For more on sleeping pills, see Chapter 6.) So if your doctor's response is to prescribe medication, you may want to proceed on your own for a while, or find a differently oriented doctor.

On the other hand, if you're concerned that your insomnia may be linked to another condition, if you're frightened by symptoms you've been having, or if you think you have sleep apnea or periodic leg movements as described in Chapter 1, you probably would do well to consult a doctor, if only to reassure yourself that your problem is "no worse than" simple insomnia. Likewise, working with a doctor or sleep specialist may help you learn more about your own particular rhythms and sleep habits. Also, if you're interested in using biofeedback to respond to your insomnia, you'll need to do so through a referral from your doctor. (For more on biofeed-back, see Chapter 6.)

A doctor who's addressing your sleep problem, whether a general practitioner or a sleep specialist, should take a thorough history of your sleep habits. Your sleep history and sleep journal give you some idea of what a physician will—or should—want to know.

If you visit a sleep center, you may be given a polysomno-graphy, a number of tests administered simultaneously while you're sleeping to measure various physical events that occur during sleep: brain function as measured by an EEG (to reveal how much deep sleep and REM sleep you're getting and to ascertain your pattern of moving through the various stages of sleep), heart rate and rhythm as measured by an electro-cardiogram, eye movement, chin movement, airflow through your nose and mouth, various aspects of your breathing, and several other functions.

A sleep specialist may also give you the Multiple Sleep Latency Test, in which your ability to fall asleep at various times of day is tested, in order to learn more about your degree of sleepiness.

Generally, enough data can be gathered in one night at a sleep center. Two or more nights is rarely necessary.

If you do choose to work with a doctor, here's what you have a right to expect:

) Courteous, respectful treatment

) Full explanations of all procedures and tests

) Full explanation of your diagnosis—why and how it was arrived at, what other possibilities are still being considered, and the like; the doctor should allow plenty of time for you to ask questions, either when you first hear the diagnosis or later, when you've had time to absorb the information

❭ Complete information about any medication that's being prescribed, including an explanation of likely and possible side effects

❭ Availability for phone calls and questions between visits, especially in response to side effects of medication; instructions about which side effects might warrant an immediate call

❭ Willingness to reevaluate treatment if necessary, and to continue a discussion with you about various options

What you in turn owe your doctor as a responsible partner in your treatment might include the following:

❭ A clear, concise description of your symptoms, concerns, and history

❭ Courtesy and respect as the two of you determine treatment together

❭ Full cooperation in carrying out any treatment plan you've agreed to

❭ Clear and accurate information of how treatment is affecting you (since subjective impressions often vary, it's usually helpful to keep a journal recording what medication you've taken and how your sleep has proceeded)

Tips for Reducing Your Time in Bed

> Cut if you will with sleep's dull knife
> The years from off your life, my friend!
> The years that death takes off my life,
> He'll take from off the other end!

> —Edna St. Vincent Millay

Even if you're struggling with insomnia or other sleep problems, you may also wish you could spend less time in bed to feel rested and refreshed. It *is* possible to reduce the amount of time in bed, but it takes discipline and commitment. If you're interested, you might consult a book called *The Sleep Management Plan: A Six-Step Plan to Add Hours to Your Week and Increase Your Energy,* by Dale Hanson Bourke. Bourke herself once "needed" eight hours of sleep to function well, but found that she could reduce her total time in bed to only six and a half hours a night. She recommends the following techniques:

1. *Assess your sleep needs and sleep patterns.* Determine what works for you about your sleeping habits and what's getting in your way: worries? physical interruptions like noise or light? Also, explore your own personal rhythms. Ideally, when would you sleep and wake? When are you most and least productive?

2. *Find out what motivates you.* Find specific activities to pursue during those extra waking hours: meditation, artistic work, exercise, time to read, an opportunity to take a quiet walk.

3. *Organize your space to support your new plans.* Make it easier to get out of bed in the morning—lay out clothes, breakfast dishes, and so on ahead of time.

4. *Create a pattern and stick to it.* Wake and sleep at the same time for three weeks, with no variation even on weekends. Then cut back one half hour every three weeks until you've reached your goal or until your daytime sleepiness alerts you to realize you need somewhat more.

5. *Choose a diet and exercise that supports your reduced sleep.* Avoid or eliminate caffeine, processed sugar and sweeteners, alcohol, cigarettes, recreational drugs, and high-fat foods. Start a regular program of aerobic exercise, thirty minutes a day, three to five times per week.

6. *Find ways to sleep efficiently.* If you can't fall asleep in twenty minutes, get up and do something else. Bourke's program may not work for everybody, but it's certainly true that many of us could get along more efficiently on far less time in bed if we led healthier lives. It's also true that the very effort to make more time for yourself may lead you to find more satisfaction in both your waking and your sleeping life.

Chapter 3

Deciphering Your Insomnia

The greatest mistake in the treatment of diseases is that there are physicians for the body and physicians for the soul, although the two cannot be separated.

—Plato

If this book were to leave you with only one message about insomnia, that message would be to remember that *your sleeping life and your waking life are one.* The temptation for many of us who can't sleep is to want to leave the problem behind in bed, to relegate it to the nighttime hours. Probably, though, the reason the problem is emerging at night is that we're not allowing ourselves to turn our full attention to it in the bright light of day.

Allowing ourselves to attend to our insomnia doesn't necessarily mean analyzing the problem. As we've seen, it's often possible to dispel our sleeplessness without ever knowing exactly where it came from.

For example, suppose you find yourself passing more sleepless nights than you're comfortable with. Rather than asking yourself why this is happening and struggling for an answer, it might simply work for you to say, "Let me try going without caffeine for a month." (For more about caffeine and sleeplessness, see Chapter 4.)

Perhaps eliminating caffeine from your diet will solve your sleep problem, even if you hadn't increased your caffeine intake at the time your insomnia set in. Maybe, too, the entire process of going without caffeine will bring you other, unlooked-for benefits—more restful sleep; fewer hours spent in bed and correspondingly, more hours spent doing things you care about; a new sense of serenity and calm; the sense that you *can* take action to improve your life. Taking action to address your insomnia may open up new possibilities in your life in a way that expands beyond the logical realm of "What's causing the problem and how do I remove the cause?"

On the other hand, it may be that your insomnia is a specific message you're sending yourself, one that won't go away until you've responded fully. Perhaps you lead a challenging, busy life, in which children, job, spouse, community involvement, and extended family all come before care for yourself. You accomplish every task you set for yourself—except the task of falling asleep. In the achiever style that works so well for you everywhere else, you set yourself some goals: to give up caffeine, to get in a brisk ten-minute walk three times a week, to cut back on sugar in your diet. But after three months, your sleeplessness persists, and you're starting to feel frantic with worry and exhaustion.

Clearly, in such a case, your insomnia requires another kind of care than you're giving it. Even in that case, however, a direct, logical, head-on approach may not be best. It may be more productive to approach the problem obliquely, intuitively, and playfully. Perhaps you need to give yourself ten minutes each night to keep a journal, in which you reflect on the events of your day. Such a process might lead you to realize that there are some changes you'd like to make in your life, changes that would indicate more respect for your limits.

Or perhaps it would help you to learn to meditate. It could be that the process of taking fifteen minutes each morning and/or evening to meditate would in itself be a useful life change, along with the actual benefits of meditation itself. Choosing to meditate might mean that you've opened up a new space in your life, one that makes room for new discoveries about your feelings, abilities, and desires. (For more about meditation, see Chapter 6.)

Rather than asking yourself, "Why am I not sleeping?" you might ask, "What do I wish I could do while I'm awake?" As suggested in Chapter 2, you might ask for a dream that would suggest a way to regain your peaceful sleep, and then reflect on the multiple possibilities that the dream raised. You might also say to yourself, "I know exactly what I need to do to regain my sleep, and that is ＿＿＿＿＿＿＿＿ ," allowing yourself to fill in the blank with a reply that may surprise you. And remember that sleep is biological function. It is something that you *let* happen, not *make* happen.

This chapter offers a number of suggestions for approaching the emotional aspects of insomnia, on your own or with a therapist. As you think about the feelings that cluster around your sleeplessness, it might be helpful to think of your insomnia not as a problem to be solved or as a disease to be cured, but rather as a message to be deciphered. Logic, analysis, and medical information might help you decode the message in your insomnia—but so might intuition, passion, and a willingness to be surprised.

Why Am I Tired?

Next to sex and hunger, the urge to sleep is nature's most powerful drive.

—Dr. William Dement

If the urge to sleep is such a powerful drive, then we have to ask ourselves what might be more powerful. When you can't sleep, what alternate need is so great, so urgent, that even the need for sleep is shoved aside?

You might try the following exercise. Find a quiet, undisturbed place where you can be alone for at least ten minutes—fifteen to thirty minutes, if possible. (If you can't imagine finding a space of ten undisturbed minutes for yourself during your day, then you might begin by exploring ways to shift your schedule or your arrangements so that some private time *is* available to you.)

Begin by choosing a comfortable position to sit or lie down in. If you choose to lie down, however, make sure that you can stay relaxed but alert—the goal for this exercise is not to fall asleep but to stay awake! If possible, try doing this exercise in silence, without background music or other distractions. You might also wish to make a tape of the following three paragraphs, or to get a friend to record a tape for you, pausing appropriately to leave you time to respond.

Close your eyes. Breathe deeply. Allow your body to become completely relaxed. Let your breath fill each part of your body. Allow your mind to wander from your head, to your face, to your shoulders, to your chest, to your arms and hands, through your tor-

so and hips, down through your legs and feet, bring-
ing relaxation to each muscle as you turn your attention to it. Continue to breathe deeply. Think of your
breath as carrying relaxation to each part of your
body.

When you feel relaxed, allow yourself to hear
the following words in your mind: "Why am I tired?
What do I need?" Whatever happens, just sit with the
question awhile, eyes closed. If you find your mind
wandering, let it wander. It may take you to an image
or a memory that will help you answer the question—
but in an unexpected way.

Continue to breathe deeply. If you feel a part
of your body tensing up, notice it and then let the
tension go. If you like, hear the questions in your
mind again: "Why am I tired? What do I need?" Let
yourself ask the questions as often as you need to.
You don't need to interpret or evaluate any of the
words, images, feelings, or other answers that might
come to you. Now is just a time for noticing.

When you've sat with the questions for a length of
time that feels right, slowly open your eyes and reach for your
notebook. Allow yourself to write whatever comes to mind—
your thoughts and feelings of the moment, what you thought
and felt while doing the exercise, or a description of another
time that has suddenly come to mind. If you feel uncertain
about what to write, put the questions at the top of the
page—"Why am I tired? What do I need?"—and then write
about whatever answers or images come to mind. If you're
having a strong emotional reaction—feeling tearful, angry,

anxious, excited, peaceful, or joyous—you might note your emotion in words or draw a picture that expresses how you feel.

It may be that this exercise produces some specific ideas for you about changes you'd like to make or particular things you now want to do. It may also be that the answers will come later, in a dream that night, or while your mind is on the grocery list two weeks later. Asking yourself this question while you're *not* in the midst of your insomnia is a way of giving the insomnia a different kind of attention and respect. It's also a way of learning how to relax while exploring your sleeplessness, rather than bending your mind to the problem in a late-night frenzy of anxiety or frustration.

Hearing the Message in Your Insomnia

Mendel found that he couldn't sleep. Tomorrow he had to move, and how could he transport his possessions to the new apartment through the blinding snowstorm coming down over the city? Then suddenly, he thought, "Goldberg can lend me his sled!" Full of hope once more, he turned to sleep—and found he was still wide awake.

"What if Goldberg won't lend his sled?" "Nonsense," he told himself. "Of course he will. Aren't I his best friend? Go back to sleep."

"But what if he won't?" "Don't be silly. I lend him money all the time. I took care of his wife when she was sick. Don't worry. Go back to sleep."

"Goldberg won't lend his sled!" "That ingrate! That two-bit chiseler! How dare he refuse me! . . ."

Mendel jumped out of bed, got dressed, and ran

down the block to Goldberg's house. When a sleepy Goldberg answered the bell, Mendel shouted, "Goldberg, you rat, you and your lousy ten-cent sled can just go straight to hell!" He left the astonished Goldberg standing in the doorway and returned home to sleep soundly at last.

—Jewish folk humor

Often when we can't sleep, it's because we feel we've left something undone or unsaid, or because we feel we need something we haven't gotten yet. Following is a list of some needs and feelings that your insomnia may be trying to express. As you read through the list, you might want to keep a journal or notebook handy. Jot down any thoughts or feelings that come to you as you read. Perhaps you'll run across a paragraph that describes exactly the way you feel; maybe you'll feel like arguing with one point or another; or perhaps something you read will inspire you to take off on another train of thought altogether. Use the list in whatever way inspires you to learn more about your own particular situation.

❭ *I need help!* Perhaps you feel uncomfortable acknowledging that you can't easily handle every challenge that comes your way. Maybe it's hard for you to admit that you need help in meeting some of your responsibilities, handling some feeling, or achieving some desired goal.

Not being able to sleep may be a way of dramatizing the problem, to yourself and/or to others, so that you can get the help you need. Having insomnia may be a way of allowing yourself to get some kind of help—even if it's for the insomnia and not for the problem that you originally wanted to solve. Or it may be a way of encouraging another person to offer you help—either specific help with a problem that your insomnia prevents you from handling, or symbolic help that reassures you of another's concern. Becoming aware of this need may enable you to ask for help more directly. It's also possible that simply *experiencing* your need for help may ease your insomnia, even if you don't act on that need.

〉 *I need time for myself.* You've got a million things to do tomorrow, and you need your sleep. Yet sleep is the one thing you can't have, because you're lying awake with insomnia. "I know I'll be a wreck tomorrow," you think in frustration. But perhaps your insomnia is a way of saying that today is more important than tomorrow. Maybe your insomnia is actually giving you a backhanded chance at having some time to yourself. Of course, there are more efficient, relaxing, and productive ways to get some private, personal time than lying awake at three in the morning. But if you aren't allowing yourself to make those other ways a priority, insomnia may be your psyche's last-ditch effort to carve out a little personal space.

〉 *I need respect for my limits.* Do you feel that you're one of the strongest, most capable people that you know? Do you often get the feeling that if you didn't do most things in your life, they just wouldn't get done? Are you the one who always takes up the slack when other people can't come through? If so, and if you're frequently struggling with bouts of insomnia, you might consider the possibility that sleeplessness is your way of staging a protest. Even as one part of yourself is saying, "Oh, that's OK, I can handle it," another part of yourself—the sleepless, out-of-control, up-in-the-middle-of-the-night part—is saying, "It's *not* OK! I *can't* handle it! Look at me—up at four in the morning, crazy with worry! Clearly, there's a problem here! Why can't someone *else* do it—someone else who's getting a good night's sleep, for example!"

The thing to remember in this case is that one part doesn't cancel out the other. Just because part of you is feeling small, lonely, and out of control, that doesn't mean your efficiency and capability are a facade or a fiction. It may mean that you purchase the image of being *always* efficient and capable at a high price, and that your insomnia is a way of dramatizing that price, to yourself and others.

⟩ *I'm angry!* It's difficult for many of us to acknowledge our anger, particularly if we feel it isn't justified. Of course, getting in touch with anger doesn't necessarily mean that we have to act on it or express it. Sometimes it's enough simply to know that we're angry. Other times, it's possible to vent our feelings to ourselves, our journals, or a friend who isn't involved, just to blow off steam. Still other times, it is helpful to express our anger or at least to assert our concerns to the person involved.

Whatever we choose to do with our anger, though, the one strategy that usually *doesn't* work is to suppress it. Insisting to ourselves that we're *not* angry, we *can't* be angry, takes an enormous psychic toll. How many times have you said to yourself, "Well, it's not that important to me," or "I'm not angry, I'm just disappointed," or "He's free to do what he wants, of course, but my feelings are a little hurt"? If these phrases sound familiar to you, you might ask yourself whether the day you said them was followed by a sleepless night. Feelings have to come out somehow, and angry feelings are no exception. If you could begin acknowledging your anger to yourself—without necessarily changing anything in your conduct with other people—you might find sleep coming more easily.

⟩ *I need sexual fulfillment.* "Going to bed" has more than one powerful meaning in our vocabularies. Whether you sleep alone, with one or more casual partners, or with a steady partner, bed connotes sex as well as sleep. And if you're not happy with what's happening in your bed, you may dramatize that unhappiness by staying up and waiting for something better.

Perhaps your sleeplessness is a silent message to your sleeping partner: "I need something you're not giving me." Perhaps it's a message to yourself. You may want to explore ways of communicating more openly with a partner, learning more about forms of sexuality that satisfy you, or changing your patterns of relationship. When you start to feel that you're taking care of this need in your waking time, you may find that sleep has returned.

❯ *I have something to tell you.* Sometimes it's unfinished business that keeps us awake. Is there a friend, family member, or loved one in your life with whom things aren't going well? Or, alternatively, is there a new love in your life, a new potential friend, or a newly appreciated family member to whom you're eager to get closer? Desires and passions—for romantic, friendly, or familial connections—can be a powerful preoccupation. Our insomnia may be a way of making space for a connection—positive or negative—that we're not fully acknowledging in our waking life.

Of course, just because we have feelings about a connection doesn't mean that we need to express those feelings to the person involved. Sometimes the best way to handle a difficult situation is to let things work themselves out. Sometimes what we most want to do with a crush or a new best friend is just to fantasize about the object of our desire, to savor the possibilities or the tiny signs of a potential mutual interest. Feeling that there's "unfinished business" doesn't have to imply that we need to finish it, or that we need to finish it *with* the person involved. We just might want to make room for that business elsewhere in our lives, so that bedtime can be spent in sleeping. Alternately, we may want to let ourselves enjoy our nighttime fantasies and simply accept that we're going to be getting less sleep for a while as a result.

〉 *I need to solve my problem.* Sometimes we're well aware that a particular problem is keeping us awake. Other times, we may experience a vague nagging feeling or free-floating anxiety without knowing which problem the feeling is attached to. In either case, we may be staying awake in order to give attention to the problem, at the expense of our sleep and our peace of mind.

If this is the case for you, you have many options. You may want to stay up late one or two nights specifically to address your problem, whatever it is. You may feel far more satisfied facing the problem out of bed when that's what you're "supposed" to be doing, rather than "sneaking" the problem into your mind when you're actually "supposed" to be sleeping. If your problem is more important to you than sleep, you might just let that be your choice and allow yourself to follow through on it.

Alternately, identifying a particular problem may free you to make time for it when it *doesn't* conflict with your sleep. Neither choice is necessarily "right" or "healthy." Either choice will probably make you feel more empowered and comfortable than wishing to sleep but not being able to.

〉 *I need more scope for my ambitions.* Is something about your work life not working for you? Are you frustrated with some aspect of your job? Do you dream—metaphorically speaking—of another type of work, paid or unpaid, a calling that would allow you to express yourself more fully, a vocation that would engage you more completely?

If so, and if you feel that your waking life doesn't allow you the scope you're looking for, you may be trying to carve a little space for your ambitions out of your sleep time. If your work dreams seem beyond your control, you may be seizing upon something that *is* within your control—your slumber. Getting in touch with your ambitions and deciding more consciously how you want to realize them might ease your insomnia.

No matter what message your insomnia is giving you, you have many options about how to hear it. You can realize that you have a feeling or a wish that you don't intend to act on. You can choose to look for a direct solution to your problem. You can allow yourself to ruminate about the problem for as long as you need to, trusting that the right answer will come to you. You might choose to get help from a counselor or friend, to write about your problem in your journal, or to handle the situation strictly on your own.

In other words, what you *do* with your new awareness is your choice—but in order to make a choice, you must first allow yourself to be aware. We frequently hide feelings or wishes from ourselves; there's nothing inherently wrong or unhealthy about doing that. Your insomnia, however, may be a sign that it's not working for you to hide some particular wish.

People often feel that once they're aware of a problem, then they must do X. They don't want to do X—so they never allow themselves to become aware of the problem. A more open-ended approach might reveal more satisfying possibilities for action. If your insomnia is "trying to tell you something," allow yourself to listen. What you do with the new information is still up to you.

Sleep and Stress

> Friedman the clothier was distressed when he learned that his partner, Weinberg, was suffering from insomnia. "Listen," Friedman suggested, "why not try counting sheep?" Weinberg agreed to try. But the next morning when he came into the store, he looked more haggard than ever. Friedman asked him what the problem was. "Didn't you try counting sheep?"
>
> "Sure, I did," Weinberg replied. "I got up to fifty thousand. Then I sheared the sheep and made fifty thousand overcoats. So far, so good. But then it hit me, and I was up all night tearing my hair—*Where was I going to get fifty thousand linings?*"
>
> —Jewish folk humor

The moral of the story is obvious: Don't take your worries to bed! Both your problems and their solutions can be distorted in the half-light of 4 A.M., and all you'll accomplish is to deprive yourself of the sleep and dream time that might actually help you solve those problems by the light of day.

Of course, that's easier said than done. But take heart. Plenty of other worriers have come before you—and they've found ways to let go, at least for a few hours. Here are some techniques that they've found helpful that might work for you, too:

❯ *Keep a journal*. Some people find that writing their problems down helps create a sense of resolution, even if they don't actually discover a solution. There's also something comforting about the journal itself—you can flip through the back pages remembering that you made it through each of those days, so why shouldn't you be all right tomorrow? Some people arrange their nighttime routine to include some journal-writing time followed by a little light reading. They find that the switch from active writing to passive reading makes a nice transition and helps them let go of their active daytime mode into a nighttime state of receptivity to sleep.

❭ *Imagine the worst.* Many former insomniacs have praised this technique for letting go of worry. They focus on the problem they're obsessing about and ask themselves, "What's the very worst that could happen?" Somehow, naming the worst takes the sting out of it, whereas letting it lurk unspoken in the back of your mind gives it a lot more power. Some people like to imagine how they'd cope with the worst, allowing themselves to relax after assuring themselves that they have solutions ready for even that. Other people find that just naming the worst makes it clear to them that their most horrible fears really aren't very likely to happen.

❭ *Make a joke.* No matter what's bothering you, if you can find the humor in it, you'll find it much easier to resolve. Allow yourself to exaggerate the situation. Find the irony in your problem, or let it remind you of a similar situation you've heard in a joke or seen on a sitcom. Nothing puts worries in perspective like laughter.

❭ *Visualize your problem differently.* Your mind is a powerful ally. Let it help you shrink your problem or remove it altogether, even if just for tonight. Picture your problem as a huge inflated balloon, and then imagine sticking a pin in it. Imagine your problem as a parcel that you place carefully in the room that's farthest from your bedroom. See yourself entering your bedroom, shutting the bedroom door, and leaving your problem outside. Picture your problem dissolving from a huge cloud into a tiny little raindrop, which you then wipe away with a towel. Or let it shrink from being a huge boulder to a tiny pebble, which you then flip carelessly out the window. You might have so much fun playing with imagery that you forget to be worried.

) *Change your self-talk.* Often a worry carries with it an underlying negative message. Beneath your apparently logical ruminations, the same idea plays over and over, like a broken record: "I'm no good"; "No one loves me"; "Only a real idiot would have this problem"; "I can't do anything right"; "If I can't fix this, then I know I'm worthless." Such negative self-talk doesn't really invite a deeper exploration of who you are and how you might improve yourself—and it certainly doesn't offer a productive way to spend your precious sleep time. See if you can allow yourself a positive self-comment: "I am loved"; "I am safe"; "I love myself"; "I have faith in you"; "I believe in you." You might also focus on positive self-talk about sleep: "I am totally relaxed"; "I am slipping off to sleep"; "I'm looking forward to my dreams"; "I feel peace."

Sleep, Sleeplessness, and Depression

I cannot forget 1895. To lie, night after night, staring wide awake, hopeless of sleep, tormented in nerves, and to realize all that was going on, when I was present, so to speak, like a disembodied spirit, to watch one's own corpse, as it were, day after day, is an experience which no sane man with a conscience would repeat.

—Lord Rosebery, British prime minister

Are people depressed because they can't sleep, or do they fail to sleep because they are depressed? The question is even more mysterious than it appears at first, because no one can agree on what actually causes depression, nor on what cures or alleviates it. We can all recognize that sense of helplessness and hopelessness, the feeling that life has lost its savor, the gloomy condition that sometimes expresses itself through tears, sometimes through numbness and apathy. We also know that insomnia and excessive sleepiness are both frequently associated with depression, and that a depressed person may sometimes suffer from both.

But the "root" cause of depression—a language for explaining and understanding it—varies widely, depending on the specialist's point of view. It's also possible that depression has many causes, or that its causes are all faces of one another, so that the various psychological and biochemical explanations of the condition are all simultaneously true.

What are some of the theories that have been advanced to explain depression? Neurologists and psychiatrists have come to believe that depression is a biochemical problem, caused by an imbalance of chemicals in the brain. The nerve cells in our brain communicate via chemicals known as *neurotransmitters*. The neurotransmitter known as serotonin seems to be involved in feelings of depression and/or well-being, as well as in headache, sleep patterns, and schizophrenia.

Support for this theory comes from the fact that tendencies to depression and migraine headache seem to run in the same families, and depression also seems to affect a person's sleep patterns. The medications known as antidepressants affect the levels of serotonin and other neurochemicals in the brain; antidepressants also tend to suppress REM sleep, which has proven to be helpful in alleviating some people's depression. (Antidepressants have also proven useful in treating migraine headache, further suggesting that sleeplessness, depression, and headache are all aspects of related biochemical disorders.)

The relationship between depression and REM sleep seems to be a powerful one, since when depressed people's sleep was reduced in certain studies, their depression, too, seemed to be alleviated. Since most REM sleep comes at the end of the sleep period, reducing a person's sleep means that REM sleep has been reduced.

Why should depression be related to REM sleep? Scientists have no idea, especially given the fact that, as we've seen, the need for some REM sleep is so strong that people go into REM rebound when they're not getting *enough* REM!

Certainly, it would seem that on a biochemical level, depression and insomnia are closely related. It also seems that what alleviates one condition will almost automatically bring relief to the other. So fortunately, it's not necessary to understand the entire complicated relationship of insomnia and depression in order to make a few recommendations that might alleviate both.

If you feel that both of these conditions are problems for you, you might try doing something counterintuitive: instead of sleeping more, sleep less. Limit your sleep to five hours a night—the amount that could contain all the deep sleep and REM sleep that you absolutely need. If five hours seems too drastic, you might choose a sleep time that you recall worked for you during a period in your life when you were not depressed, or experiment with gradually reducing your sleep time half an hour every two to three weeks.

If this idea appeals to you, it's crucial that you support this effort in the ways described at the end of Chapter 2, all of which are in any case useful for combating both depression and insomnia: get regular aerobic exercise; reduce or eliminate your intake of caffeine, sugar, and high-fat foods; avoid all alcohol and recreational drugs; and keep to a regular sleep schedule. You might also review your prescription medications with your doctor, eliminating any that are not absolutely necessary or exploring the possibility of reducing dosages. Avoid all over-the-counter medications, even aspirin or other painkillers, whenever possible; many have added caffeine or other elements that militate against sleep. And absolutely avoid any type of sleeping pill, whether over-the-counter or prescription: any type of sleep aid tends to suppress both deep sleep and REM sleep, so that reducing your total hours of sleep might then deprive you of types of sleep that you actually need. (*Be sure to see your doctor before making any changes in your use of prescription sleeping medications.* For more on sleeping pills in general, see Chapter 6.)

If you're interested in this approach, you'll probably want to give it a month or so. Don't reduce your sleep all at once, and allow time for yourself to feel changes in diet and exercise.

It's also significant that L-tryptophan, a chemical found in turkey and other foods that seems to help people sleep, is used by the body to manufacture serotonin. So to combat both sleeplessness and depression, you might also eat plenty of foods with L-tryptophan. (For more on L-tryptophan, see Chapter 4.)

Even if the idea of reducing your total sleep time doesn't appeal to you, you might consider approaching both depression and insomnia by getting exercise and modifying your diet. Meditation (explored further in Chapter 6) has also proven helpful in alleviating both insomnia and depression.

Few people of whatever viewpoint would disagree that diet, exercise, and meditation are helpful tools in overcoming depression, insomnia, and a host of other conditions. But those who view depression as primarily an emotional illness might point out that restructuring your life and adopting a new healthy regime is precisely what seems so out of reach when you're depressed. People of this view would argue that, even if depression can be viewed as a biochemical event, its sources are primarily psychological; therefore, a primarily psychological approach to both depression and insomnia is needed.

Different schools of psychology interpret depression differently. Generally, however, those in the psychoanalytic tradition believe that depression represents suppressed anger, grief, and other feelings that the depressed person believes are not safe to feel or are somehow "bad." If people believe that their true feelings of helplessness, anger, resentment, or despair will somehow hurt themselves or others, they'll have a powerful reason to hide those feelings from themselves—but those hidden feelings may then emerge as depression. Believing that our feelings are "bad" is something we learned in childhood, so these beliefs also tend to exist on a primitive, hidden level. By definition, we're not conscious of feeling that way, but psychoanalysts would argue that both depression and persistent insomnia are clues that our minds and bodies are trying to give us, clues to something we're not yet willing to

know consciously. Many people who have undergone psychoanalysis agree that once they became aware of their grief and
anger, their depression lifted, and with it, their insomnia.

Analysts stress that becoming aware of buried feelings doesn't necessarily mean acting on them. A person may
realize that, say, she's been angry with her father all her life,
without then needing to express that anger directly to her father. Likewise, a person might realize that he has felt unloved
by his parents in important ways while also realizing that his
parents cared for him and did the best they could. But, an analyst would say, fully experiencing the buried feeling will release a person from the depression—as well as from the
insomnia that might accompany it.

Jungian analysts have a somewhat different view of
depression. They tend to view it in mythic terms, as a natural
part of human growth and development. A Jungian analyst
might see depression as a stage that comes just at the point
when a person is ready to make a big life change, passing
from one era of life into another. Depression in this view is an
experience to be mined and learned from. Once the lessons
of a particular depression have been learned, the depression
will pass. In this view, too, a person with insomnia might seek
to hear the message in the insomnia rather than proceeding
immediately to "cure" the sleeplessness.

If either of these perspectives appeals to you, you
might consider seeking a therapist who can help you explore
one of them more deeply. (See below for more information on
therapies that are available along with some suggestions on
how to find them.)

Seeking a Therapist

> Our sleep can be undisturbed only if we are free from tension and sure of the solution of our problem.
>
> —Alfred Adler

There is certainly a great deal you can do on your own to explore the emotional issues that may be feeding your insomnia. But you may decide that, in the long run, you'll get further working with a partner—a therapist, counselor, or psychoanalyst who can help you explore themes and issues in your life more deeply and who can provide you with an alternate perspective. Although therapy doesn't guarantee solutions to your problem, to paraphrase Adler, it does insure that you'll have help in finding the solutions that are right for you.

Therapeutic help is available in a wide variety of forms. Some therapists might focus specifically on overcoming your insomnia. Others might believe that the insomnia is only a clue inviting you to look at deeper issues. Among both groups, you might find practitioners with a wide range of approaches. To help you choose the philosophy that's most congenial to you, here are brief descriptions of some of the major types of therapy and psychoanalysis that are available:

❭ *Short-term therapy.* When we think of "therapy," we tend to think of a long-term process, but short-term or "brief therapy" lasts several weeks at most. If you want to focus only on your insomnia, this is probably the type of therapy that you're looking for, as short-term therapy tends to be organized around a specific problem that the patient wishes to solve.

Often a therapist and patient will make a contract, specifying what the problem is and what the patient would consider a satisfying solution—a solution that the therapist believes can be achieved in a relatively short amount of time.

The advantage of short-term therapy is that it allows you to focus on a particular problem with relatively little expense or time commitment. The disadvantage is that it may leave many key issues in your life unexplored, so that either the insomnia or some other symptom may continue to reappear.

) *Behavioral therapy.* Behaviorists usually aren't interested in *why* people have problems; they're more interested in altering behavior so that the problem goes away. A behaviorist might address your insomnia by helping you to establish a regular sleep schedule, for example, assisting you in finding out what would reinforce your ability to stick to that schedule and helping you discover how you can discourage yourself from breaking it. The advantage of behavioral therapy is that it's often quite effective in solving a particular problem. Its disadvantage is that, in failing to look at the feelings and psychological history that created the problem, it opens the door for the problem to reemerge, perhaps in another form.

) *Cognitive therapy.* Often, it's our ideas about the world that get in our way. Believing that the world is a hostile place, that nice guys finish last, or that good girls put others first may be assumptions so deeply ingrained that they shape our behavior without our realizing it. Cognitive therapy seeks to help patients become aware of their preconceptions and assumptions, and to replace counterproductive cognitions (understandings) with ideas that allow for more satisfaction. The advantage of cognitive therapy is that it tends to be very concrete: patients often feel a sense of liberation in discovering how their own thoughts are holding them back, along with excitement about seeing the world in a new way. The disadvantage of this approach is that if you have a deep emotional stake in believing a certain precept, it may take more than a cognitive (rational) understanding to help you change that belief.

) *Modern analysis.* This school of therapy is closest to the thinking of Sigmund Freud, the founder of psychoanalysis, although many changes have occurred in the field since its inception a century ago. Modern analysts tend to focus on what they see as a person's basic drives toward sex and aggression; one of their major goals is to encourage patients to get in touch with the full range of their feelings. As we've seen, "getting in touch" with feelings doesn't necessarily mean expressing them. Rather, it means letting go of the guilt, fear, and shame that many people attach to having "bad" feelings of helplessness, anger, or unacceptable desires. In a sense, the lesson in modern analysis is "Despite what you've come to believe, your feelings aren't dangerous to yourself or to others. Rather, even your 'bad' feelings can be a source of enormous energy, wisdom, and joy once you learn to accept them." The advantage of modern analysis is that it attempts a profound exploration of a person's deepest feelings. Its disadvantage is that it can be a costly process that often lasts for several years, requiring a huge—though potentially rewarding—commitment of time and energy.

) *Self psychology.* Self psychology shares much in common with modern analysis in that it is a long-term exploration of feelings rather than a short-term approach to a specific problem. Whereas modern analysis focuses on drives that may have their dark side, self psychology tends to stress the positive aspects of human emotion. Where a modern analyst might speak of a patient's rage, for example, a self psychologist might refer to the person's deep need to be heard and understood. The advantage of self psychology is that it presents a somewhat more positive image of human emotion than other schools of psychoanalysis tend to do. The disadvantage is that in focusing on the positive, it may inadvertently encourage patients to continue feeling ashamed of emotions they perceive as negative.

) *Jungian analysis.* The followers of psychoanalyst Carl Gustav Jung also engage in long-term psychoanalysis, but their work goes in a somewhat different direction from that of either modern analysts or self psychologists. Jungians tend to look for the mythic aspect in all things, relating an individual's preoccupations to the cultural stories that reveal similar preoccupations throughout the ages. Where a modern analyst or self psychologist might focus on a particular incident in which a father humiliated his son, for example, the Jungian analyst might encourage the patient to explore what the notion of "fatherhood" means to him, using myths and cultural images of "father" to expand his ideas about his family, his role, and himself. Jungians also rely heavily on a patient's dreams, which they see as revealing a person's deepest preoccupations as well as connecting individuals with our mythologies. The advantage of Jungian analysis is that it can be a rich and open-ended means of exploring issues in one's life, providing a spiritual dimension often lacking in the other schools of therapy. The disadvantage is that patients may feel that their individual stories get somewhat lost in the mythic worldview.

If you'd like to find a therapist but aren't sure how to go about it, you might ask a friend for a referral, approach a religious leader for advice, or look for advertisements in publications you enjoy reading. Other suggestions might come from a doctor or another type of health practitioner. Social service agencies listed in the Yellow Pages can usually refer you to a therapist as well.

You may know exactly the type of therapy you're looking for—or you may want to shop around. It's perfectly acceptable to make initial appointments with several therapists in order to determine which you'd finally like to see. Of course, you'll probably have to pay for each appointment, but many therapists offer discounts for a first session.

A first session is often a time when the therapist may ask you questions, as he or she tries to find out more about who you are and why you've come. Even at first, however, a good therapist should do more listening than talking. Nor will a good therapist jump in and try to solve your problem for you; he or she may not even offer any advice. Rather, a therapist is supposed to help you identify your own problems and come to your own solutions. The therapist's job is to provide insight and perspective, based on his or her philosophy.

You may wish to use some of your first session to ask the therapist questions. It's usually not appropriate to focus on your therapist's personal life—marital status, children, and the like. However, it's quite appropriate to ask about the therapist's philosophy and to hear what he or she thinks you'll get from the therapy. It's also appropriate to ask how long the therapy may take, to go over fee and insurance arrangements, and to find out the therapist's policy on scheduling, makeup sessions, and missed sessions.

Your best guide to choosing a therapist is ultimately your own intuition. Do you feel respected and listened to? Do you feel that the therapist sees you as an individual, or as just another example to be fit into a predetermined slot? Does the therapist seem to be on your side while still letting you be responsible for your own problems and solutions? Do you have the feeling that this is someone of integrity, someone whom you could come to trust?

In our individualistic culture, it's often difficult to ask for help. The process of seeking and choosing a therapist may itself be therapeutic, as we start to understand that we're not alone and that there are resources out there that can support us. Just knowing that you don't have to solve all your problems alone can make you feel better, even before you've found the person with whom you want to work. Finding a challenging and supportive therapist may turn out to be one of the unexpected benefits of deciphering your insomnia.

Chapter 4

Feed Yourself to Sleep

> *"You feel sleepy, don't you, my dear?" said the doctor.*
>
> *"No, sir," replied Oliver.*
>
> *"No," said the doctor with a very shrewd and satisfied look. "You're not sleepy. Nor thirsty. Are you?"*
>
> *"Yes, sir, rather thirsty," answered Oliver.*
>
> *"Just as I expected, Mrs. Bedwin," said the doctor. "It's very natural that he should be thirsty— perfectly natural. You may give him a little tea, ma'am, and some dry toast without any butter. . . ."*
>
> —Dickens, *Oliver Twist*

Today's sleep specialists would have mixed feelings about the efforts of Oliver's doctor to help his young patient get some sleep. The dry toast is probably a good idea. Toast—especially if it's whole-grain—is rich in complex carbohydrates and B vitamins, both potent dietary sleep aids. And leaving off the butter means that little Oliver's stomach won't be burdened with any hard-to-digest fats, so that his system is left free to focus on sleep.

On the other hand, the caffeine in the tea might keep the young patient from feeling sleepy for quite some time.

And if Oliver takes his tea with sugar, as many people do, his system will get an additional buzz that might keep him up even longer.

Which foods help bring on sleep and which keep sleep at bay? As with all questions relating to insomnia, there are no easy answers, partly because the experts don't always agree, partly because every sleeper's body functions differently. One woman might drink two cups of coffee ten minutes before bedtime with no noticeable ill effects; another can't sleep if she has a single cup with breakfast that morning. A man might find that a dish of yogurt or a glass of hot milk sends him off to sleep without fail, while his brother discovers that his system rebels against all dairy products, particularly those taken at bedtime.

In this chapter, you'll find information about how diet affects your sleep. Some of the opinions presented here will be unanimous. For example, virtually everyone agrees that caffeine, sugar, white flour, additives, and preservatives militate against sleep. Likewise, it's generally accepted that people with sleep problems should avoid nicotine, alcohol, and recreational drugs.

Other opinions will be in conflict. For example, most Western doctors feel that sleep is aided by a low-fat diet, while Deepak Chopra, M.D., trained in both Western medicine and in the Ayurvedic medical tradition of India, holds that oily foods help bring on sleep. People from a wide range of traditions favor dairy products as sleep aids, but macrobiotic theories of diet claim that dairy products are difficult to digest, a difficulty that interferes with sleep even as their calcium calms the nerves and their L-tryptophan induces slumber.

To find your way through the thicket of conflicting views, use your own judgment, and rely on your intuition. Everyone's body is different, and what affects most people one way may affect you quite otherwise.

It's also important to remember that food is a potent emotional trigger. Sure, a glass of warm milk contains calcium and L-tryptophan—but to many of us, it also signifies *Mother, comfort,* or *childhood security*. Likewise, a fragrant cup of coffee isn't just a caffeine-loaded, sleep-destroying beverage—it may also represent a beloved ritual, a special "private time," or a delicious accompaniment to a favorite meal.

As we examine which foods nurture or destroy our sleep, we always need to take our emotional associations into account. Otherwise, we'll be operating on incomplete information, not fully able to take the actions that will truly work for us.

How Food Affects Our Sleep

Your foods shall be your remedies, and your remedies shall be your foods.

— Hippocrates

As we've seen throughout this book, the causes and the cures of our insomnia are not always symmetrical. In some cases, our diet might be said to cause our insomnia; in other cases, diet may be only one contributing factor among many; in still other cases, diet may be relatively neutral in its effects. Nevertheless, in all three situations, changes in diet may be immensely beneficial in restoring restful sleep, even if diet wasn't the primary cause of the insomnia in the first place.

There are many ways in which our diet affects our sleep patterns. Most nutritionists believe that insomnia is integrally related to an imbalance of proper nutrients in our bodies. Poor nutrition leads to difficulties *digesting* and *metabolizing* food—that is, to trouble breaking food down into vitamins, minerals, and other essential nutrients, absorbing them, and rearranging their molecules. A well-nourished body digests and metabolizes easily, deriving nutrients, creating energy, and eliminating waste. A poorly nourished body may experience distress in the process of digestion and metabolism, and it won't get the maximum benefit from the foods it processes. It may signal nutritional deficiencies or excesses with all sorts of complaints—migraine headaches, gas pains, excess weight, high blood pressure, a general sense of tiredness and/or depression, and, of course, sleep difficulties.

To better understand how food interacts with our bodies, let's look at the digestive process step by step.

As soon as you take a bite of food, the enzymes in your saliva start to break the food down. You swallow, and the partially broken-down food flows into your esophagus, a long tube that carries the food into your stomach. Chemicals in the stomach break the food down further, until it reaches its final destination—the small intestine. At this point, the food has been broken down into nutrients—protein, carbohydrates, vitamins, minerals, fat—and waste. The nutrients pass into your bloodstream through the small intestine's wall, so that the blood can carry each nutrient to the body part that needs it. Bones, muscles, tissue, and nerves are all renewed as the blood carries nourishment to them.

The waste, meanwhile, passes into your large intestine, and eventually, into your rectum, which expels it regularly. In some cases, though, waste rots or decomposes within the large intestine before passing into the rectum. If this happens to you, you'll experience it as indigestion, perhaps accompanied by gas pains. And if you've ingested anything that the body experiences as toxic—say, additives, preservatives, artificial coloring, or the artificial hormones frequently added to meat and chicken—your large intestine will be additionally burdened by the extra toxins.

Just as nutrients pass into the blood through the small intestine, so do toxins enter the blood from the large intestine. And just as the blood carries nutrients throughout the body, it transports toxins to the liver, whose job it is to purify the blood.

As you can see, your liver has quite a job to do. Clearly, it's an easier job if you're eating only pure, natural, and low-fat foods. Imagine, then, how the liver's work increases with each toxic addition to your diet: additives and preservatives, rancid oil (found in many snack foods), fatty foods, alcohol, nicotine, and caffeine. Recreational drugs create additional liver strain by depositing yet more toxins into the bloodstream. Although there may be good reason to take prescription medications, the liver experiences these as toxic also.

Clearly, digestion requires a great deal of energy from the body. It involves several organs—stomach, small intestine, large intestine, and liver. In addition, the kidneys process liquid wastes in the form of urine, and the pancreas secretes insulin to process the blood sugar metabolized from the food you've eaten. (For more on the role of blood sugar in insomnia, see below.) As you visualize the digestive process, you can see how what you eat determines whether digestion proceeds smoothly or with difficulty. Certain foods—particularly those with a high fat content—are harder to digest. Other foods—particularly those high in animal protein—are more likely to decompose while still in the large intestine. Still other foods contain toxins that strain the liver.

Nutritionists believe that these digestive difficulties drain the body of energy. That's why a meal high in animal protein (particularly beef, pork, and other high-fat meats), fats, and toxins is likely to leave a person feeling tired and logy. That's also why many people report new surges of energy when they switch to a healthier diet. Their bodies are working far less hard to derive nutrients from the food ingested. The healthier diet is also designed to contain enough of the nutrients that each body part needs, so that every part of the body is far more likely to be well nourished.

By the same token, digestive difficulties can interfere with sleep. The body has to work extra long and hard to digest certain types of food, particularly those high in fat or toxins. This prolonged hard work militates against restful sleep. That's why eating high-fat foods, smoking cigarettes, or drinking alcohol before bedtime may either keep you awake or produce fitful, unrefreshing sleep. Your body is literally at odds with itself. (The nicotine in cigarettes and the sugar in alcohol may also serve as stimulants, and alcohol interferes with sleep patterns; for more on their particular effects, see below.)

Some nutritionists focus on teaching their clients which foods the body needs and which strain the body, as well as helping each individual client find the particular mix of nutrients that's right for him or her. Other nutritionists rely more heavily on vitamin and mineral supplements, arguing that foods today are so likely to be stripped of their essential nutrients that we can no longer rely on nature alone to provide us with what we need.

You might want to explore working with a nutritionist of either type to learn more about your particular metabolism and nutritional needs. You may discover that you've been operating on shortages of certain essential vitamins, minerals, or other nutrients—perhaps even of the very elements that help promote restful sleep. (For more on these elements, see below.) You might also use the information in this chapter to experiment with your own diet. Through a combination of intuition, study, and experiment, you may come up with a diet that both eases your digestion and nourishes you more efficiently. If so, you've probably taken a big step toward overcoming your insomnia.

Blood Sugar, Diet, and Insomnia

> THE SOLDIER: I've no ammunition. What use are cartridges in battle? I always carry chocolate instead. . .
>
> — George Bernard Shaw, *Arms and the Man*

Shaw meant his soldier's remark to be ironic, but in fact he was hitting upon on an important truth. Chocolate, like all other sweets, plays a crucial role in the rise and fall of our blood sugar. But the same chocolate that helps the soldier endure the rigors of battle may also play havoc with his ability to enjoy a good night's sleep.

To understand how diet and blood sugar might affect our rest, let's look again at the digestive process. We've already seen how both nutrients and toxins pass into the bloodstream. One of these nutrients is glucose, or blood sugar.

Despite the sweet name, glucose is processed from a number of different foods, including such high-protein foods as milk, cheese, meat, and fish, and from such complex carbohydrates as whole grains. Glucose levels in the body rise most quickly, however, when you've eaten something sweet or something made from processed white flour.

Glucose is extremely important to our sense of energy and well-being. That's why, if you're tired and hungry, you often feel better right after you eat—your blood-sugar levels have gone back up. And, as we'll see in a moment, a shortage of glucose—low blood sugar—can make you feel dizzy and irritable and can interfere with memory and concentration.

Generally, after a meal, your body has absorbed more nutrients than you can use right away. But the human body has an ingenious system for holding on to excess nutrients. It stores some as body fat (which causes weight gain) and stores others in the liver as glycogen, a substance that can be converted easily into glucose as needed.

Blood sugar is one source of your body's energy and sense of well-being, for it passes from the blood into your body's tissues. That's one reason why any part of the body that is cut off from circulation will, in effect, die: it isn't getting the nutrients—including the blood sugar—that it needs.

Because blood sugar is so crucial to survival, your body is always trying to keep its blood sugar at a certain level. Inevitably, though, blood sugar rises and falls. When you digest food, your blood-sugar level rises. Your body responds by producing *insulin*, the substance that moves blood sugar out of the bloodstream. Then the blood-sugar level falls. When it falls far enough, you'll feel hungry, eat some more, and start the whole process over again.

Diabetes, or *chronic hyperglycemia*, is a disease in which a person's pancreas is unable to produce or release enough insulin to utilize blood sugar. Instead of passing into the body, blood sugar remains within the diabetic's blood. If this condition isn't corrected by the administration of insulin from another source or other drugs, the diabetic can die.

However, some people have the opposite condition—*hypoglycemia*. In this condition, an overactive pancreas produces too much insulin, so that blood sugar falls too quickly. As we'll soon see, hypoglycemia may be a trigger for insomnia.

Many doctors deemphasize the role of nutrition in various conditions, and so they tend to recognize only a strict definition of hypoglycemia. This standard medical definition is based on a person's reaction to a five-hour glucose tolerance test. The tested person is fed and then told to fast for the next five hours as his or her blood-sugar level is periodically tested. A healthy person's blood sugar will go up immediately after being fed, then decrease gradually over the next five hours as nutrients pass slowly from the blood into the rest of the body.

A diabetic also experiences a rise in blood sugar after eating—but his or her blood sugar levels will then remain abnormally high for at least two hours. As we saw, a diabetic's blood sugar isn't being processed by insulin, so the nutrient isn't leaving the blood for other body parts. Blood sugar stays high while body parts "starve."

A hypoglycemic, on the other hand, will experience a drop in blood sugar well before the normal five hours after eating—and sometimes as quickly as only two hours after eating. Moreover, a hypoglycemic's blood sugar drops to far lower levels than that of a healthy person. After a healthy person eats, his or her normal pancreas eventually lowers blood sugar down to 70 to 100 mg (milligrams) percent (per 100 milliliters of blood). But after a hypoglycemic eats, his or her overactive pancreas quickly lowers blood sugar down to 40 to 50 mg percent. In other words, blood sugar rushes out of the blood into other body parts at a rate that is too fast.

As we've said, this is the standard medical definition of hypoglycemia, as determined by the glucose tolerance test. However, many nutritionists recognize a milder version of the condition known as *relative hypoglycemia*. The following symptoms characterize relative hypoglycemia: feeling anxious, irritable, depressed, moody, or confused after missing a meal; losing memory or concentration after missing a meal; feeling dizzy, having tremors, or breaking into a cold sweat after a missed meal; continually craving sugar or sweets; feeling that once you start eating sweets, you can't stop; getting a headache when a meal has been missed or delayed.

If these symptoms sound familiar, you might want to explore how diet may be involved in your insomnia, even if your condition doesn't show up on any tests. If your diet is high in sweets, processed white flour, alcohol, caffeine, and/or nicotine, you may also be creating conditions in your body that mimic hypoglycemia—and these conditions may be interfering with your sleep.

To understand how diet relates to sleep, we have to go back to what happens when you eat something sweet or starchy. Eating foods made with processed sugar or white flour infuses a huge amount of glucose into the system very quickly. This confuses the pancreas, which produces even *more* insulin—to drive blood sugar down even more quickly. If you've ever felt a sugar "high" and then a sugar "crash," you've experienced the dramatic effects of rising and falling blood sugar levels.

Sugar and processed white flour aren't the only substances that drive up your blood sugar. Caffeine, tobacco, marijuana, alcohol, and cocaine produce drastic increases in the blood-sugar level, which is why these substances tend to take away your appetite: they've fooled your body into thinking that it has already eaten, because your blood-sugar level has gone up. (The inhaling of marijuana is eventually followed by an enormous increase in appetite, but its initial effect is to dull hunger.) That's also part of why a stimulated high tends to be followed by a crash—once your blood-sugar level goes up dramatically, it's likely to fall just as suddenly.

What actually happens when your blood sugar level has a sudden drop? Your body experiences this process as a severe emergency. Even though you've just eaten, you may experience symptoms that resemble those of someone who is literally starving: anxiety, irritability, panic, inability to concentrate, trouble with memory, and possibly a feeling of faintness, dizziness, or light-headedness. (These are also the symptoms a diabetic experiences if he or she takes insulin and then doesn't eat.)

Of course, you're *not* starving. But the body knows only two states: safe—a normal level of blood sugar; and in danger—a low or high level of blood sugar. The body doesn't know how to distinguish between blood sugar that's low because it has already been utilized, and blood sugar that's low because the person hasn't eaten for days.

When the body experiences an emergency, it responds by triggering one of our oldest survival mechanisms, the "fight or flight" reaction. Through a complicated process of hormonal interactions, your body mobilizes to meet the perceived emergency: body temperature rises, as do blood pressure and pulse rate, breathing becomes shallower, and you feel anxious, keyed up, alert, and ready for danger.

Thus, if you've eaten something sweet or starchy just before bedtime, or if you've smoked a cigarette, had a few drinks, or driven your blood sugar up in some other way, you may find your sleep disturbed. Depending on what you ate and when, you may find yourself in the middle of a blood-sugar high or low just as you're trying to fall asleep. Both the "wired" feeling of unnatural energy that accompanies the high and the panic reaction that goes with the crash make it harder for your body to enter into that state of relaxation necessary for slumber.

Alternatively, like many insomniacs, you might find yourself easily able to fall asleep only to awaken in the middle of the night, overwhelmed with exhaustion and anxiety. Perhaps you wake suddenly, with a pounding heart, rapid breathing, and furiously racing thoughts. At such times, you might look for psychological reasons to explain your reaction—but perhaps you're also reacting to the sudden drop in blood sugar.

Do any of these patterns sound familiar to you? If so, you might want to explore your eating habits with a nutritionist, to see how your diet might be modified to help improve your sleep. Or you might want to try out the following guidelines, adjusting and experimenting as you find out what works best for you:

) Avoid processed sugar in all its forms: granulated and powdered sugar, honey, maple syrup, corn syrup, and dextrose. Be vigilant about reading labels, because corn syrup and dextrose are added to a surprising number of packaged, processed, and frozen foods, even to food items that we don't normally consider sweet. Honey is also deceptive, as bees are often fed processed sugar or corn syrup. Likewise, stay away from such sweet foods as cookies, cakes, ice cream, and candy.

) Reduce or eliminate the following foods which, although not as sugary as most desserts, nonetheless will place a strain on your metabolism of blood sugar: soft drinks, juices or beverages with added sweeteners (again, that's most of them), canned or frozen fruit, baked beans, baked goods, dates, raisins, and dried fruits.

) Avoid the following foods that are made from white flour, as that, too, converts very quickly to glucose: potato chips, pretzels, and novelty snacks like Chee-tos.

) Focus on moderate amounts of high-protein foods such as lean meats, fish, and poultry; dairy products; soybeans and related foods, such as tofu and miso soup; nuts, seeds, and unsweetened peanut butter. Proteins metabolize to glucose slowly, so that they help the pancreas produce less insulin, so that you don't experience a sudden crash.

) Focus also on relatively large amounts of healthy foods such as green leafy vegetables; other vegetables; and fresh fruits. Remember, though, that fruits of all kinds contain sugar, however natural. Depending on how sensitive you are, you may find that it's better not to eat fruit on an empty stomach or just before bedtime.

) Some starchy foods are less sweet than others. Whole grains, whole-grain bread, pasta (even white pasta), and potatoes are generally acceptable except for the most extreme hypoglycemics. However, whenever possible, combine a starchy food with a protein or a fat. That will help slow down your digestion, blunting the effect of the starch on your blood sugar. (If you must eat sweet foods, you might also try combining them with a protein, too, such as drinking a glass of milk with your dessert.)

⟩ Think about the timing of what you eat. If you're having trouble sleeping, and if you recognize hypoglycemic patterns or symptoms from this description, you might try to eat fruits and starches earlier in the day, so that your blood sugar levels are calm by bedtime. Some naturopaths (doctors who focus on nutrition and theories of natural foods) advise patients to cut out sweet foods entirely and to eat fruits and starches only before 2 P.M.

⟩ Generally, try to eat small, regular meals rather than large, infrequent ones. Extreme hypoglycemics must eat every two hours to keep their blood sugar steady. Even relative hypoglycemics get uncomfortable when they've missed a meal, however. Make sure you have some protein at every meal.

⟩ Eliminate any beverage or food that contains caffeine: coffee, tea, colas, chocolate. Decaffeinated coffees also tend to contain small amounts of caffeine. Depending on your sensitivity, you might avoid caffeine in all its forms, or again, drink only small amounts earlier in the day. Of course, ingesting caffeine is a bad idea for problem sleepers anyway. (For more on caffeine, see below.)

⟩ Don't be fooled by so-called "natural" desserts that are nevertheless loaded with sweeteners. A whole-wheat carob cookie sweetened with honey is far more likely to trigger a hypoglycemic reaction than plain old white spaghetti or a baked potato, especially if you've put cheese on the spaghetti or butter on the potato.

❭ Likewise, avoid artificial sweeteners. While these won't trigger a hypoglycemic reaction, they may be unhealthy for other reasons. Many studies have linked saccharine to cancer, while aspartame (found in NutraSweet and Equal) may decrease the body's serotonin levels which, as we have seen, regulate sleeping patterns as well as depression, headache, and our general sense of well-being. Moreover, artificial sweeteners seem to increase people's craving for the real thing.

❭ Depending on your rhythms, you may need to avoid all late-night eating. On the other hand, some hypoglycemics need to eat a light snack, such as crackers and a mild cheese, just before going to bed, so that their blood sugar won't fall during the night. In extreme cases, hypoglycemics might set their alarms in order to wake up and eat a small protein snack during the night.

❭ If you do wake up with late-night panic reactions, and you think their source might be a blood-sugar problem, see if a high-protein snack helps calm your system. A low-fat food will be easiest to digest: no-fat milk, cottage cheese, or yogurt; a little tuna fish on whole-wheat bread; or just a glass of skim milk.

The Benefits of Water

He who drinks much water after meals will never suffer from stomach trouble.

— Jewish folk saying

Folk wisdom may be putting the case a bit strongly, but it's perfectly true that drinking several glasses of water per day is one of the healthiest things you can do for yourself. As we've seen, your blood carries toxins from the food you've digested, as well from the alcohol, nicotine, and other substances you've taken into your system. Your blood also carries away metabolic wastes and other toxic material that your body produces on its own.

Therefore, keeping yourself well hydrated increases the volume of blood and helps flush out the toxins. It eliminates waste from your system without draining away essential nutrients, which is why drinking large quantities of water is often recommended for people trying to lose weight.

If you can, try to drink eight glasses of water a day—a total of two quarts. You may be surprised at how much better you feel after such a simple change. Be extra sure to drink a glass or two of water before exercising: toxins are often stored in body fat, and vigorous physical energy that burns up the fat also releases the toxins.

Water is also a good antidote to other sleep-destroying substances. If you've had a few drinks, if you smoke cigarettes, or if you've eaten a high-fat dinner, water can help counteract these substances' antisleep effects.

You might want to stop drinking a couple of hours before bedtime, particularly if you find yourself frequently waking up at night to use the bathroom. On the other hand, you should drink lots of water *after* you ingest alcohol, nicotine, or large quantities of fat, so if you've up been late partying, water will probably ease your sleep, even if you do have to get up once or twice during the night.

Deepak Chopra recommends another way of drinking water that he says is highly valued in the Ayurvedic tradition. According to Dr. Chopra, hot water helps dissolve impurities in the body. In his view, what's important is not the total amount of water ingested, but rather the frequency: he suggests taking a sip or two of hot water every half hour if possible, or at least every hour or so. He recommends water so hot that you have to blow on it before you can drink it.

People who want to try drinking large amounts of cold water might try to keep a plastic water bottle with them at work, so that they can pour themselves a glass or two once or twice an hour. Those who wish to try Dr. Chopra's recommendation might fill a thermos with boiling water, which should stay hot for up to ten hours.

In either case, you may find yourself urinating much more often if you're not used to drinking water frequently or in large quantities. Some people find this process discomfiting, while others say it makes them feel healthier. In either case, you'll probably feel it most intensely when you first start your new water regime, as this is the time when many toxins are being flushed out of your system. As you get used to drinking more, your system will calm down again.

The Problem of Salt

> Since food vendors face cutthroat competition, there are no holds barred when it comes to enhancing taste. And the cheapest way to hook the consumer is by adding salt.
>
> — Douglas Hunt, M.D., *No More Cravings*

Like sweeteners, salt is added to virtually every packaged, processed, and frozen food that you can buy. Yet for the person with sleep difficulties—as for people with headaches, high blood pressure, and many other chronic conditions—salt may be one of the worst items you can eat.

Salt stimulates the nervous system, which certainly tends to interfere with sleep. It increases the accumulation of fluids in the body, which tends to increase blood pressure. It also interferes with the elimination of some waste products as your body metabolizes food. Although the ill effects of salt can to some extent be counteracted by drinking water to flush the salt out, it's best if you can radically cut down or even eliminate salt from your diet.

Dr. Michael M. Miller of St. Elizabeth's Hospital in Washington, D.C., experimented with reducing the salt intake of twenty-five patients in his care. Those in the study showed a marked improvement in ability to fall asleep—sleep onset time declined to only fifteen minutes. Most went on to sleep soundly through the night. Yet when the doctor increased the salt in the diets of thirteen of these patients, without their knowledge, ten of them resumed their sleep problems within only a few days.

If you're interested in reducing your salt intake, you'll have to put a certain amount of effort into eating fresh foods that you prepare yourself. Restaurants habitually add large amounts of salt to their offerings, as do food manufacturers of a wide range of foods. Frequently, low-fat desserts, salad dressings, and similar products make up the lost flavor from the missing fat by increasing salt, so read the labels carefully.

You may find that saltless food tastes bland to you at first. Take heart—if you can stick out your new regime for about ten days or so, you'll find that suddenly your palate has become far more sensitive to all sorts of new flavors. Meanwhile, you might compensate by eating foods that are naturally high in salt, such as uncooked fruits and vegetables, nuts, seeds, and seafood. You might also turn to other spices—but use moderation. Spicy foods can stimulate your system and interfere with digestion, which will in turn disturb your sleep.

The Perils of Caffeine

Using spiders, scientists at NASA labs in Alabama have identified the chemical agent responsible for human error. . . . Anyone who has ever had a tip from an excitable stockbroker go south, or had the rearview mirror fall off his brand-new car when he slammed the door and discovered it was made on the night shift. . . will be struck by the slipshod, disorderly, ill-planned, chaotic, and slaphappy structure laid down by the spider intoxicated by caffeine. It's the construction of a lonely man laboring in the middle of the night in a room at the Insomnia Hotel, his head bent over a piece of paper, and a neon sign outside his window endlessly repeating "SLEEP, WORK, SLEEP, WORK."

—"Talk of the Town," *The New Yorker*

It's hard to credit the sleep-destroying properties of caffeine. After all, so many of us drink coffee, tea, and cola, so many of us eat chocolate. Each day, more than 400 million cups of coffee are drunk in America alone, a great many by people who claim that they need this beverage in order to wake up.

It's ironic that coffee has the reputation of a wake-up beverage, because it actually makes you more tired. Certainly, the initial ingestion of caffeine produces a big lift—but that lift is soon followed by a crash, requiring yet another cup of coffee (or some other stimulant, like a cigarette, a cola drink, or something sweet to eat) to straighten us out.

Remember the way that drastic ups and downs in blood sugar might affect sleep? Well, caffeine relies upon that reaction—and intensifies it. Caffeine stimulates your "fight or flight reaction," helping the body to mobilize itself for an emergency. Among other things, it stimulates the adrenal glands to produce hormones that in turn tell the liver to convert glycogen into glucose, raising your blood-sugar level quickly. If you lived in a prehistoric village, you might need this extra burst of energy to face down a ravening beast, or to run quickly away from danger. In that case, your physical exertion would quickly burn up the excess blood sugar.

But if you're not facing a physical challenge of that magnitude, your blood-sugar level remains high. You feel tense, keyed up, and ready for an emergency that isn't coming—until your pancreas releases the insulin that will burn up the excess blood sugar and, often, bring on a postcaffeine crash.

These ups and downs can be exhausting. Furthermore, caffeine remains in the body a long time, frequently interfering with the restfulness of sleep. People who have given up caffeine report that in about two weeks to a month they are sleeping more deeply and efficiently. In many cases, they're able to get along better on less time in bed.

Caffeine taken near bedtime will probably have the greatest impact on the length and quality of your sleep. The more caffeine you drink and the closer to bedtime you drink it, the more likely you are to be deprived of REM sleep, and the more difficulty you'll probably have in falling asleep and staying asleep.

Sleep specialist Dr. Quentin Regestein says that caffeine's effects peak two to four hours after ingestion, and that you may feel the effects from two to seven hours after drinking. Other sleep experts cite an even longer time: twelve to twenty hours. Thus, an after-dinner, afternoon or even morning cup of coffee can still plague you at bedtime.

Caffeine appears not only in beverages and in chocolate but in many popular medications as well, as this chart demonstrates:

CAFFEINE IN YOUR DIET

Source	Estimated Caffeine in Milligrams
Brewed coffee—1 cup (five ounces)	100–150
Instant coffee—1 cup	85–100
Decaffeinated coffee—1 cup	2–4
Tea—1 cup	30–40
Cocoa—1 cup	40–55
Chocolate bar	25
Cola—8 ounces	40–60
Anacin	32
Bromo Seltzer	32
Cope	32
Darvon compound	32
Excedrin	65
Midol	32
Vanquish	33

If you decide you'd like to reduce or eliminate caffeine from your diet, here are some suggestions:

> If you're prone to headaches, you may not want to go cold turkey. Caffeine tends to constrict the blood vessels, so that when the effects of the caffeine wear off, the blood vessels expand too quickly, causing headache pain. Cut down by half a cup every other day, meanwhile increasing your intake of calcium and B vitamins.

> As you reduce or eliminate caffeine, make sure you're getting plenty of protein to counteract the effects of "lost" caffeine on your blood-sugar levels. Without the artificial stimulus of caffeine, your blood sugar may feel unusually low more often than you're used to. Regular, small, high-protein snacks; vigorous aerobic exercise; and avoiding alcohol will all help you make it through the "withdrawal" period.

> Consider replacing one or two cups of a caffeinated beverage with a similar, noncaffeinated beverage. Although the chemicals used to decaffeinate some coffee and tea are harmful in other ways, they probably won't affect your sleeping patterns (except insofar as they tax your liver—like any other toxin!). Cafix, Postum, Pero, and other natural-grain beverages can feel almost as satisfying as coffee or tea, particularly if you take milk in your hot drinks. Many people find herbal teas soothing and satisfying.

> Be careful not to increase your consumption of sugar as you switch beverages. Both caffeine and processed sweeteners can give your blood sugar a lift—but, as we've seen, that artificial burst of energy is ultimately bad for your sleep.

> Discover some alternate treats for your coffee or tea breaks. What's the point of making your diet healthier if you

feel that you're enjoying your life less? Perhaps it's feasible to take a brisk walk in a pleasant spot, or to snatch ten minutes with a favorite book or magazine. Maybe you can substitute fresh fruit for your caffeinated beverage—treat yourself to mangoes, strawberries, or some other special food that you normally wouldn't indulge in. Be creative in your search for ways to be good to yourself.

Alcohol, Nicotine, and Recreational Drugs

> She'd take a little gin for her nervousness, then a little for her tiredness. . . .
>
> — John Cheever, "The Sorrows of Gin"

It may be difficult to associate alcohol with wakefulness, since our usual image of someone who drinks too much is that he or she passes out. Yet alcohol actually interferes with sleep in a number of ways. Acutely, it suppresses REM sleep, which, as we've seen, can sap the restorative powers of sleep. Chronically, it tends to reduce the amount of deep Stages 3 and 4 sleep. People who drink frequently and/or have a dependence on alcohol tend to wake during the night, as they switch from one sleep cycle to the next. Often they "medicate" these wakeful periods with another drink to induce sleep, further destroying the restful quality of their slumber.

Insomnia may also be a side effect of withdrawal from alcohol. In fact, a heavy drinker may experience withdrawal during the night, which may also lead the person to wake up needing a middle-of-the-night drink.

People who are addicted to nicotine and cocaine may experience a similar effect, waking up in withdrawal. Certainly, when a person is trying to quit smoking or stop using cocaine— as well as other drugs, both stimulants and sedatives—insomnia can be a potent and painful side effect. A doctor's care may be needed in treating the insomnia that can result from the withdrawal process.

In any case, as we've seen, nicotine and cocaine are both stimulants, as are amphetamines and some other recreational drugs. As stimulants, they make it difficult to sleep during the "high" periods.

Marijuana is not physically addictive, but it does alter the chemicals involved in sleep and changes the brain-wave patterns. It seems that long-term use of marijuana can increase the time it takes for a person to fall asleep—an effect that may be exacerbated if a steady user makes a habit of smoking before bed to relax. A person who has developed such a habit may find it more difficult to fall asleep *without* smoking. In addition, marijuana also suppresses REM sleep, making sleep after smoking less restorative.

Calcium

> Calcium can be as soothing as a mother, as relaxing as a sedative, and as life-saving as an oxygen tent.
>
> — Adelle Davis

Calcium is truly a natural sedative. Found in dairy products, eggs, leafy green vegetables, and seaweed, it calms the nervous system. It also helps the sleep center in the brain to function. Think of the soothing properties of a glass of warm milk at bedtime, and you can picture the relaxing properties of calcium.

Insufficient calcium is likely to leave a person feeling both tense and fatigued. Women who are premenstrual tend to be low on calcium; the premenstrual time is also often an emotionally tense time, as well as a week marked by sleep disturbances.

According to Dr. H. C. Sherman of Columbia University, 50 percent of all U.S. residents are not getting sufficient calcium. Adelle Davis also thought Americans were calcium-starved, a condition that she thought was closely linked to insomnia. She used to recommend that her insomniac patients take a couple of calcium tablets with a milk drink at bedtime, and to drink milk and take tablets during each subsequent hour that their sleeplessness continued.

An alternative way of taking calcium is to drink a quart of milk enriched with half a cup of powdered milk. Or you might drink buttermilk made from skim milk, since the acid helps the bloodstream to absorb the calcium in this form. Davis recommended four glasses of buttermilk and lots of yogurt to those who had sleep problems.

Other calcium-rich foods include cauliflower, broccoli, figs, oranges, almonds, soybeans, and blackstrap molasses. Powdered animal bone—bone meal—is also a good calcium source. (It can be purchased at health-food stores.)

If you are interested in getting calcium through dairy products, you should probably try to stick to skim milk and low-fat cheese as far as possible. The fat in whole-milk products may strain your digestion and make sleeping more difficult, in addition to causing you other problems.

Many nutritionists discourage their clients from eating dairy products, even if the people aren't technically lactose-intolerant (unable to digest milk). If so, you can see that plenty of alternative calcium sources are available to you. Don't get sidetracked by constant references to "warm glasses of milk." Make sure that, through supplements or natural foods, you're getting enough of this essential mineral.

In order to absorb calcium efficiently, your body also needs magnesium. Most nutritionists believe that few adults are getting more than about half the minimum daily requirement. White flour, sugar, and even small amounts of alcohol destroy magnesium, so even if you're consuming foods that contain this mineral, you may be deficient in it.

Magnesium is available in food supplements, as well as in sea salt, kelp, all kinds of seeds, nuts, beets, spinach, dates, and prunes.

L-*tryptophan and the* B *Vitamins*

> "Hannah," said Mr. St. John at last, "let her sit there at present, and ask her no questions; in ten minutes more, give her the remainder of that milk and bread. . . . "
>
> A kind of pleasant stupor was stealing over me as I sat by the genial fire.
>
> — Charlotte Brontë, *Jane Eyre*

There's that warm milk again! It's no wonder that milk keeps showing up in writings about sleep, because, in addition to being rich in calcium, it contains another natural sedative, L-tryptophan. This amino acid appears naturally in a great many foods, including meats, fish, poultry, eggs, dairy products, nuts, soybeans, and other high-protein foods, contributing to the sedative qualities of large meals.

According to researcher Dr. Ernest Hartmann of Boston City Hospital, one gram of tryptophan cuts down the time it takes to fall asleep by ten to twenty minutes, as well as increasing subjective sleepiness—the individual's sense that he or she wishes to sleep. (As we'll see in Chapter 5, subjective sleepiness and objective sleepiness—one's actual readiness to sleep—don't always link up.)

Tryptophan seems to be involved in the production of serotonin, the neurotransmitter involved in sleep disorders as well as in depression and migraine. (For more about serotonin, see the section on depression in Chapter 3.) In experiments on cats, for example, extreme reductions in serotonin levels have prevented the animals from sleeping for several days.

Unfortunately, tryptophan is no longer available as a supplement because of its linkage to a blood disorder, eosinophilia myalgia syndrome, in 1989. Many of the two hundred victims of this disease had been taking L-tryptophan supplements, so authorities banned the product from the market, and so far, it hasn't reappeared.

Most sleep specialists agree that L-tryptophan itself was not the culprit, but some foreign substance that presumably entered during the packaging process. Previous to the scandal, L-tryptophan had been prescribed and administered in moderate doses for twenty years without incident, and tryptophan is still widely used for treating depression in Great Britain with virtually no reports of any side effects at all.

If you can't buy L-tryptophan as a supplement, you can increase its occurence in your diet. Logically, you might assume that increasing your protein intake would boost your tryptophan levels, but actually, that isn't the case. Although high-protein foods *are* high in tryptophan, they're also high in other amino acids, substances that will compete with the tryptophan for space on the "carrier molecules" that transport amino acids to the brain.

A high-carbohydrate diet, on the other hand—plenty of whole grains (especially oatmeal) and pasta—along with such tryptophan-rich foods as green peas, spinach, lima beans, cashews, peanuts, and peanut butter, is more likely to help you sleep. Why? The carbohydrates stimulate the production of insulin (as we saw earlier, in the section on blood sugar). Carrier molecules are free to carry L-tryptophan into the brain, where it can produce serotonin.

You can test this for yourself: are you sleepier after eating a high-protein meal or after one high in carbohydrates? Probably the protein helps wake you up (which is why it's good to eat high-protein meals earlier in the day) and the carbohydrates help calm you down (which is why carbo-rich meals should be eaten around dinnertime—but not too late!).

If you really want to make sure that tryptophan is being properly used by your body, be sure you're getting enough vitamin B_6. Apparently, this essential B vitamin is key to the absorption and use of tryptophan, as well as contributing generally to the reduction of stress.

Actually, all of the B vitamins help to reduce stress, which is another good reason for people with sleep disorders to take B-vitamin supplements and to eat foods rich in B vitamins, such as organ meats, fish, whole grains, wheat germ, walnuts, peanuts, bananas, sunflower seeds, yeast, dairy products, and blackstrap molasses.

Interestingly, caffeine destroys B vitamins—while increasing stress. Stress also destroys B vitamins, so those of us with high-stress diets can both relax more easily and sleep better if we up our intake of B vitamins.

Here are just a few examples of how the B vitamins help us cope:

) B_3, niacinamide, seems to be involved in raising the serotonin level. It has also proven useful in treating hyperactive children, being particularly effective in helping them sleep.

) Deficiencies of B_6, pyridoxine, seem to cause weight loss, irritability, apathy—and insomnia. B_6 seems to be a sedative, calming substance, and it has been used to treat palsy, St. Vitus's dance, and epilepsy. It helps maintain magnesium levels (which in turn helps us use our calcium) and seems essential for the proper functioning of the brain. Birth-control pills destroy B_6, so if you're taking oral contraceptives, you might consider supplements of this vitamin. B_6 in your system also decreases dramatically with age.

) Pantothenic acid is used to convert sugar and fat into energy, as well as to help cells function generally. It's particularly important to the workings of the adrenal gland, and therefore is integrally involved in hypoglycemia; even in relative hypoglycemics, low blood sugar tends to stimulate an adrenaline rush as the body mobilizes to meet the "emergency." Thus, pantothenic acid is also a useful anti-insomnia substance.

) B_{12} seems to be helpful in treating depression and insomnia.

) Inositol, a B vitamin also found in citrus fruits, has been used as a natural sleep aid.

If you think you're suffering from a B vitamin deficiency—and most people are, unless they've taken specific steps to prevent it—you might consider either supplements or a daily dose of brewer's yeast, the most concentrated natural form of B vitamins. Most people can't stand the taste of yeast, but debittered yeast mixed with juice, yogurt, or cereal is certainly edible, and you may be amazed at how upping your B-vitamin intake affects not only insomnia but also hypoglycemia, stress, general energy level, and headache.

Traditional and Folk Remedies

> Breakfast like a king, each lunch like a rich man, and eat dinner like a poor man.
>
> — Traditional folk saying

There's more than a grain of truth—no pun intended—in the old folk wisdom that advises high-protein meals for earlier in the day and the poor person's portion— whole-grain bread and maybe a little milk—for the end of the evening. As we just saw, carbohydrates stimulate the transport of tryptophan to the brain, which helps in turn to stimulate sleep. And as we saw earlier in this chapter, proteins are harder for the body to digest, so they're best digested early.

In Ayurvedic nutrition, foods to help combat insomnia would include dairy products; oils; rice and wheat (but not barley, corn, millet, buckwheat, rye, or oats); oranges, bananas, avocados, grapes, cherries, peaches, melons, berries, plums, pineapples, mangoes, and papayas (but not apples, pears, pomegranates, or cranberries); beets, cucumbers, carrots, asparagus, sweet potatoes, and some peas, leafy vegetables, broccoli, cauliflower, celery, zucchini, and potatoes (but no sprouts or cabbage); nuts of all kinds (but few beans, except tofu); chicken, turkey, and seafood (but no beef or pork). Chopra recommends hot breakfast cereal for dinner, as well as such starchy foods as pasta, minestrone soup, or a dish of rice and buttered lentils.

Other cultures have their recommendations to combat insomnia. The Pueblo Indians recommend mushrooms. The Chinese make a mixture of chopped ginseng and orange peel, mixed with honey. A Gypsy remedy consists of lettuce cooked in a half-pint of boiling water with a little salt. Another, more appetizing recipe is the Gypsy mixture of lemon juice, orange juice, two tablespoons of honey, and hot water; they also recommend hot grapefruit juice. In Scotland, oatmeal gruel with honey is the preferred sleep cure, while Vermonters mix three tablespoons of apple cider vinegar with a cup of honey, taking two teaspoons at bedtime and, if necessary, two more teaspoons an hour later. People in the Balkans favor buttermilk half an hour before bed. Other folk remedies include a raw onion on toast at bedtime, a teaspoon of olive oil taken with the evening meal and a second teaspoon before bed, and a mixture of malted milk, olive oil, and hot water taken no less than an hour before bed.

If any of these remedies sound appetizing to you, it can't hurt to experiment. You may be reacting to a deficiency of an essential vitamin or mineral, some essential element that the folk remedy may offer.

Generally, as you think about your diet and insomnia, following your instinct is probably the best guide you have.

Once you've learned how digestion works and what vitamins and minerals you need, experiment—in moderation—with what you've learned. Your own sense of relief when you remedy a deficiency or cut out a stimulant will help you know that you're on track.

Chapter 5

Time Is on Your Side

*In the point of rest at the center of our being, we
encounter a world where all things are at rest . . .*

— Dag Hammarskjöld

For the millions of preindustrial years that made up
most of human history, people's lives were lived according to
the rhythms of nature. Lacking safe, reliable, or cheap ways
of making light, they mainly went to bed when it got dark and
got up with the sun. In many cultures, people slept long
hours in winter and few hours in summer. They organized
their lives around growing seasons, around the cycles of hot
and cold, rainy and dry.

But even in those unmechanical days, nature's
rhythms weren't the only ones people lived by. Human beings, like all mammals, come equipped with their own biological clocks, a cluster of cells in the hypothalamus that
actually keeps time for us. (This "biological clock" has nothing to do with the popular notion of a time by which a woman
has to get pregnant.) Long before human beings discovered
standardized time, long before we invented the first sundials
and hourglasses and pocket watches, people were living according to an inner timekeeping system that we have in common not only with other mammals but with virtually every
other living thing, including single-celled algae.

Our internal clocks control a wide variety of rhythms that must function in some way independently of external conditions if we are to survive. Rhythms whose cycle extends for longer than a day are known as *infradian rhythms*, such as the monthly menstrual cycle. (Animals who hibernate by season are also operating on infradian rhythms.) Rhythms whose cycles last less than a day are known as *ultradian rhythms*; these include our heartbeats, our breathing, and the electrical activity in our brains. The ninety-minute REM-NREM sleep cycle is also an ultradian rhythm.

And of course, rhythms that take approximately twenty-four hours to complete are known as *circadian rhythms*, from the Latin words *circa* (around) and *die* (day). The sleep-wake cycle is a circadian rhythm, as are the rhythms that govern our metabolisms, fluctuations in our body temperature, and the release of hormones and other biochemicals into our system—all of which affect our sense of being tired or alert.

Although internal clocks control our rhythms, they also exist independently of them. That is, our bodies have an inborn sense of such rhythms as breathing, heartbeat, and menstruation. But our bodies can also "tell time" for us, sensing how much time has passed or knowing how to recognize the same time each day, in a way that is independent of the regularity of rhythmic cycles.

If you think about how fickle external cues can be, you can see why all living things need their own inborn sense of time. As Harvard University sleep researcher Martin Moore-Ede explains, an animal whose feeding area is approximately two hours away from its nighttime shelter has to have its own inborn sense of what two hours is, so that it can be sure to leave early enough to get home before dark. If it were running on external cues only—say, the angle of the sun—one rainy day could throw off its whole sense of timing. You might say that the function of an internal clock is to liberate a creature from the whims of nature.

On the other hand, since external cues *are* constantly changing, our internal clocks can always be reset. This is true for most living creatures, more so as you go up the evolutionary scale, and most so for human beings. People are remarkably adaptable creatures—therein lies our evolutionary strength, in our ability to make tools, build shelters, and otherwise adapt ourselves to a wide variety of conditions. So human rhythms have both their own internal logic and a wide range of receptivity to external cues.

How does this affect your ability to fall asleep? Quite profoundly, as it turns out. Many people's sleep problems come from too many changes in their sleep patterns, such as shift workers who must adapt to night work but try to be awake with their families on weekends and holidays. Others develop insomnia by "practicing" staying up late for several days—say, to meet a deadline, or in response to stress—and then find it difficult to set back their clocks to earlier bedtimes. Still others follow the dictates of their internal clocks—only to find that their clocks run on a schedule that in no way matches the orderly nine-to-five world around them.

On the other hand, many people, no matter what the source of their insomnia, find great benefit in learning to stick to a regular sleep schedule. Going to bed and getting up at the same time day after day enables many people to spend less time in bed as well as to sleep more productively, feeling better rested and happier with both their waking and their sleep time. Many people, too, learn to use naps as a way of going with their internal rhythms of sleepiness and alertness.

In this chapter, you'll learn more about what circadian rhythms are and how they work. And you'll find some suggestions for tuning into your own unique rhythms, so that you can make the most of every minute on your biological clock.

The Power of Circadian Rhythms

> The world is as we are.
>
> —Ayurvedic saying

The first modern verification of circadian rhythms was made in 1729 by French scientist Jean Jacques d'Ortous de Mairan. He got to wondering about why plants opened their leaves during the day and closed them during the night. Were they responding to the sunlight's external cues? He put a plant into a dark room and observed. To his amazement, the plant's leaves opened anyway, suggesting that the plant's rhythm was governed not by the sun but by an internal clock.

Thirty years later, Mairan's compatriot Henri-Louis Duhamel supported the notion of an internal clock by demonstrating that plant behavior was likewise independent of external variations in temperature. In 1832, the botanist Augustin de Candolle made another fascinating discovery: not only were plants running on their own internal clocks, but those clocks were set to a twenty-two-hour cycle. In other words, although the plants he studied did have a "daily" schedule, their day seemed intriguingly free of Earth's twenty-four-hour day.

Later scientists discovered that in fact, different species do have "days" of different lengths, ranging from twenty to twenty eight hours. Nocturnal animals seem to have biological days that are somewhat shorter than twenty four hours. Diurnal animals, like humans, tend to have days that are longer. We now know as well that some humans' inborn "days" are longer and/or more irregular than others'.

In 1929, German scientists discovered that creatures can use their inborn clocks to create new rhythms. They left out food for bees at specific times, and gradually the swarms came to feed "by the clock." Later the scientists stopped leaving food—but the bees continued to show up at mealtime. Apparently, even creatures as low on the evolutionary ladder as bees can use their internal clocks to make autonomous decisions about time.

Bees continued to be a source of fascinating discoveries for scientists. The original German experimenters discovered that in order for the insects to learn the mealtime, food had to be offered no more nor less than once every twenty-four hours. Leaving food at longer or shorter intervals didn't seem to work—the bees' clock apparently ran on a twenty-four-hour schedule.

The Germans repeated the experiment in an underground mine, where the bees had no external cues to help them determine time. Nevertheless, as long as the food was left at the same time each day, the bees could learn to come and get it—and they kept coming at that time even after the food was no longer there.

In 1955, French scientist M. Renner trained bees to feed between 8 P.M. and 10 P.M., French time. Then he took the bees to New York City. The next day, the bees were still feeding between 8 P.M. and 10 P.M.—French time. Undisturbed by jet lag, the bees' internal clocks were still operating on their own time, clearly responding to an inner sense of time rather than to any type of external cue in light, temperature, or the like.

Scientists speculated that bees needed their steady clocks to keep up with the opening and closing times of flowers, on whose nectar they depended. As we saw, flowers open and close according to their own schedules, and bees had to be able to learn and respond to those schedules if they were ever going to extract nectar from the flower.

Twentieth-century scientists have engaged in all sorts of experiments to assure themselves that biological clocks operate on their own autonomous logic, rather than in response to subtle external cues. In one study, researchers took hamsters, fruit flies, and fungi all the way to the South Pole. There they spun the creatures on a table counter to the earth's rotation. Even this departure from normal conditioning didn't seem to affect the operation of the creatures' internal clock.

Circadian Rhythms and Human Sleep

> The tendency of mankind when it falls asleep in coaches is to wake up cross; to find its legs in the way; and its corns an aggravation.
>
> —Dickens, *Martin Chuzzlewit*

Even in Dickens's time, travel seems to have disrupted sleep. In our own time, when "coach travel" takes us across time zones, we've come to appreciate how radically modern technology disrupts human circadian rhythms.

Modern notions of time have changed so drastically that it's hard to realize that the world ever operated without standardized time. Only a little over a hundred years ago, each U.S. community made its own decisions about what time it was. A town might be only a few miles away from its neighbor—yet its high noon could be several minutes earlier. Thus San Francisco's clock was set over three hours earlier than that of New York City—and four minutes earlier than that of nearby Sacramento.

Railroads were one of the first technologies to help standardize time, because they were the first means of travel to regularly cross time zones. After years of negotiations and arguments among meteorologists and other experts, the railroads finally won the establishment of Standard Time. To mark the occasion, on November 18, 1883, a ball was dropped in the heart of New York City—starting a tradition that's still followed every New Year's Eve. No longer would Sacramentans and San Franciscans tell time according to their own natural relationship to the sun. Although it took many years for every state and city to agree, a standardized notion of time had been created.

Meanwhile, another new technology was beginning to render irrelevant humanity's old relationship to sunlight. In 1879, Thomas Edison had invented the electric light, giving humanity the power to turn night into day. Although gas and oil lamps had been available before Edison's discovery, people couldn't really read—or work—by such light for long periods of time. Even the poet Emily Dickinson, a notorious night owl, preferred to compose in total darkness rather than to use gaslight.

With the advent of electricity, however, cities began to expand their system of streetlights. Illuminated advertisements and well-lit nightspots changed the face of urban life, at the same time that an expanding industrial economy was drawing more and more people into cities and away from the countryside.

If the human sleep-wake cycle operated inexorably on a certain schedule, the availability of a compelling nightlife would have been irrelevant. People would find themselves feeling sleepy when the sun went down, no matter what tempting occupations might be available by artificial light. But as late-twentieth-century experiments revealed, the human sleep-wake cycle can be notoriously *ir*regular. This means that we have many options about when to sleep and wake—but it also means that there are more opportunities for insomnia and other sleep problems.

Just how irregular is the human sleep-wake cycle? Several experiments have found that just as plant and animal cycles diverge from the twenty-four-hour day, so do those of humans. A number of studies have isolated people from external cues—in underground caves, bunkers, and sleep laboratories—to discover that most human clocks run on a twenty-five-hour cycle. Left to our own devices, then, our "natural" rhythms would not fit the regularity of an industrialized lifestyle, where most of us must be at our posts at the same time every morning.

Not only does the human cycle not conform to the twenty-four-hour day, but it also tends to be rather malleable in any case. Experiments in which people have been isolated for up to six months from all external time cues—no clocks, no social contact with outsiders, total control over light levels—reveal that after a point, people's schedules tend to become irregular. Frequently, people will run on very long biological days, for thirty five to fifty hours at a time, interspersed with twenty-five-hour days. In either case, total sleep time expands or contracts, so that it constitutes about one-third of the "day."

Irregularity of sleep-wake times also seems to occur spontaneously under these conditions. Each day, people in the experiment would go to bed an hour or so later than the day before, waking up a corresponding hour or so later the next "morning." This progressively later bedtime would continue until the experimental subjects were completely out of phase with the rhythms of the outside world. Of course, as the people kept moving ahead an hour at a time, sooner or later, they would move back into phase—but then, eventually, they'd go out again, as their free-running schedules defied all conventional notions of "appropriate" sleep-wake times.

Since there were no external time cues to correct them, the people in these studies were not aware of being out of phase, of course. They were only doing "what came naturally," and in fact, they reported feeling more alert than usual.

From these studies, scientists have concluded that we rely on what they call *entrainment*. Left to themselves, our internal clocks will not spontaneously conform to a regular schedule of any kind. During the preindustrial era, of course, our clocks were *not* left to themselves. The light during the daylight hours served as a powerful source of entrainment.

But the inventions of the electric lightbulb and the continuously moving assembly line created both work and leisure that could be undertaken as easily at night as during the day. Today late-night television, brightly lit bars and restaurants, global telephone conferences, international stock market quotations, coast-to-coast faxes, and a host of other developments all create powerful reasons—counterentrainment, if you will—to operate around-the-clock.

As a result, many of us lose a sense of both the world's rhythms and our own. There is no strong, regular external environment—the rising sun, the community rituals—to keep our internal clocks in line. At the same time, we can't afford to let our clocks run free, going to bed an hour later each day until we're eventually sleeping from, say noon to 8 P.M. The modern industrialized world requires regular schedules even as it helps to make them difficult.

Night Owls and Larks

> Cleo and I would have our coffee out on the back porch every morning and watch the sun come up and listen to the birds . . . we'd always have about three or four good old hot cups of Red Diamond coffee and toast with peach or green pepper jelly, and we'd talk. . . .
>
> — Fannie Flagg, *Fried Green Tomatoes*
> *at the Whistle Stop Cafe*

Does Flagg's description of a sunrise breakfast on the back porch appeal to you? Or does the whole idea sound like something you could do only if you'd been up all night?

If you feel that you "naturally" gravitate toward early morning hours, sleep-research slang would dub you a lark. Late-nighters, on the other hand, are known as owls.

Which one are you? Take the following quiz (taken from *Wide Awake at 3:00 A.M.: By Choice or by Chance?* by Richard M. Coleman) and find out.

OWL AND LARK QUESTIONNAIRE

Instructions:

1. Please read each question very carefully before answering.

2. Answer *all* questions.

3. Answer questions in numerical order.

4. Each question should be answered independently of others. Do *not* go back and check your answers.

5. All questions have a selection of answers. For each question place a cross alongside *one* answer only. Some questions have a scale instead of a selection of answers. Place a cross at the appropriate point along the scale.

1. Considering only your own "feeling best" rhythm, at what time would you get up if you were entirely free to plan your day?

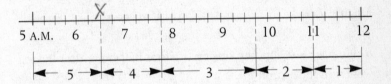

2. Considering only your own "feeling best" rhythm, at what time would you go to bed if you were entirely free to plan your evening?

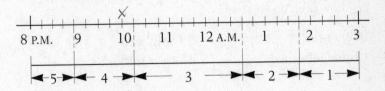

3. If there is a specific time at which you have to get up in the morning, to what extent are you dependent on being awakened by an alarm clock?

4 Not at all dependent   3 Slightly dependent
2 Fairly dependent   1 Very dependent

4. Assuming adequate environmental conditions, how easy do you find getting up in the mornings?

1 Not at all easy   2 Not very easy
3 Fairly easy   4 Very easy

5. How alert do you feel during the first half hour after having woken in the mornings?

1 Not at all alert   2 Slightly alert
3 Fairly alert   4 Very alert

6. How is your appetite during the first half hour after having woken in the morning?

1 Very poor   2 Fairly poor
3 Fairly good   4 Very good

7. During the first half hour after having woken in the morning, how tired do you feel?

1 Very tired   2 Fairly tired
3 Fairly refreshed   4 Very refreshed

8. When you have no commitments the next day, at what time do you go to bed compared to your usual bedtime?

4 Seldom or never later   3 Less than one hour later
2 One to two hours later   1 More than two hours later

9. You have decided to engage in some physical exercise. A friend suggests that you do this one hour twice a week and the best time for him is between 7 and 8 A.M. Bearing in mind nothing else but your own "feeling best" rhythm, how do you think you would perform?

4 Would be in good form   3 Would be in reasonable form
2 Would find it difficult   1 Would find it very difficult

10. At what time in the evening do you feel tired and, as a result, in need of sleep?

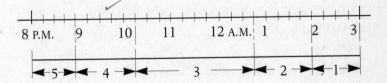

11. You wish to be at your peak performance for a test that you know is going to be mentally exhausting and lasting for two hours. You are entirely free to plan your day, and considering only your own "feeling best" rhythm, which one of the four testing times would you choose?

6   8 to 10 A.M.   4   11 A.M. to 1 P.M.
2   3 to 5 P.M.   0   7 to 9 P.M.

12. If you went to bed at 11 P.M., at what level of tiredness would you be?

0 Not at all tired

5 Fairly tired

2 A little tired

9 Very tired

13. For some reason, you have gone to bed several hours later than usual, but there is no need to get up at any particular time the next morning. Which one of the following events are you most likely to experience?

4 Will wake up at usual time and will *not* fall asleep

3 Will wake up at usual time and will doze thereafter

2 Will wake up at usual time but will fall asleep again

1 Will *not* wake up until later than usual

14. One night you have to remain awake between 4 and 6 A.M. in order to carry out a night watch. You have no commitments the next day. Which one of the following alternatives will suit you best?

2 Would *not* go to bed until watch was over

1 Would take a nap before and sleep after

3 Would have a good sleep before and nap after

4 Would do all sleeping before watch

15. You have to do two hours of hard physical work. You are entirely free to plan your day. Considering only your own "feeling best" rhythm, which one of the following times would you choose?

4 8 to 10 A.M.

2 3 to 5 P.M.

3 11 A.M. to 1 P.M.

1 7 to 9 P.M.

16. You have decided to engage in hard physical exercise. A friend suggests that you do this for one hour twice a week and the best time for him is between 10 and 11 P.M. Bearing in mind nothing else but your own "feeling best" rhythm, how well do you think you would perform?

1 Would be in good form   2 Would be in reasonable form
3 Would find it difficult   4 Would find it very difficult

17. Suppose that you can choose your own work hours. Assume that you worked a five-hour day (including breaks) and that your job was interesting and paid by results. Which consecutive hours would you select?

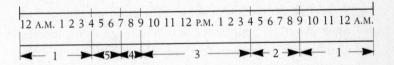

18. At what time of the day do you think that you reach your "feeling best" peak?

19. One hears about "morning" and "evening" types of people. Which one of these types do you consider yourself to be?

6 Definitely a morning type
4 Rather more a morning than an evening type
2 Rather more an evening than a morning type
0 Definitely an evening type

Scoring For questions 3, 4, 5, 6, 7, 8, 9, 11, 12, 13, 14, 15, 16, and 19, the appropriate score for each response is displayed beside the answer.

For questions 1, 2, 10, and 18, the cross made along each scale is referred to the appropriate score value range below the scale. For question 17 the most extreme cross on the right-hand side is taken as the reference point and the appropriate score value range below this point is taken.

The scores are added together and the sum converted into a five-point morningness-eveningness scale: 61

	Score
Definitely morning type	70–86
Moderately morning type *Most*	59–69
Neither type *People*	42–58
Moderately evening type	31–41
Definitely evening type	16–30

In fact, researchers are unsure to what extent the night owl/lark distinction is simply a popular perception and to what extent it represents actual biological tendencies. Research seems to suggest that only about 20 percent of the population is extremely predisposed in one direction or the other. Most people are "moderately" morning or evening, according to the scale, which means that they can shift their schedules, if need be, with some success. People who are "neither" have a very easy time shifting their schedules, whereas people who fall into that 20 percent of the population who are hard-wired have a harder time functioning well outside of "their" time.

Night owl or lark tendencies seem to have something to do with another circadian rhythm—the daily fluctuation of body temperature. Scientists have long known that there's a strong correlation between the rise and fall of body temperature and periods of feeling alert or sleepy. Generally, under normal entrained conditions, falling body temperature is associated with falling asleep, and during sleep, temperature seems to drop even more sharply.

This correlation is supported by studies that have shown that poor sleepers' temperatures *don't* drop—or don't drop enough—just before and during sleep. In one study, people who said they slept poorly had higher body temperatures than self-described good sleepers from two hours before they fell asleep to about four hours afterward. Sleep researcher Mortimer Mamelak further discovered that poor sleepers' temperatures generally stay higher throughout the night than that of good sleepers. He suggests that the energy expended by the body in keeping the temperature high militates against the potential restfulness of sleep.

However, there are many times during our daily cycle when sleepiness and temperature don't coincide. Most people feel sleepy twice during the twenty-four-hour day: before an evening bedtime but also sometime during the afternoon. Many people nap—or wish they could nap!—during this time; indeed, many cultures have established an afternoon "siesta" time as part of the normal workday. Yet the midafternoon increase in sleepiness seems to occur just as body temperature is approaching its daily high point.

It's also true that when subjects are allowed a free-running sleep-wake pattern, as in the experiments described above, the relationship between body temperature and sleep-wake cycles breaks down after about a month. The temperature cycle's ups and downs seem to settle into a twenty-four- or twenty-five-hour day, while the sleep-wake cycle, as we saw, may expand into days of as long as thirty-five to fifty hours.

Moore-Ede concludes from this that we have at least *two* biological clocks, one that governs sleep-wake cycles, another that governs temperature. Entrainment—establishing a regular sleep-wake pattern—helps synchronize the two cycles, so that the temperature cycle reinforces our sleep-wake rhythms.

In other words, like the bees that showed up for the same daily feeding time, maybe we've developed a conditioned response. We feel our body temperature drop—and we automatically begin to feel sleepy. You can see why that would be a useful bit of conditioning. If we waited for our sleep-wake cycle to determine our bedtime, we'd go to bed an hour later each night. Our nighttime temperature, however, falls at pretty much the same time each night. If we condition ourselves to respond to that signal, we'll tend to feel sleepy at the same time each night—and our sleep-wake patterns will stay in synch with the rest of the world.

You can also see why establishing regular sleep and wake times is so important, especially for people who have trouble falling asleep. That's because our sleep-wake cycles by themselves won't establish any kind of regularity for us— they need to be supported with external cues.

In fact, it's remarkable how little our subjective sense of "feeling sleepy" may correspond to the times our body is actually ready to fall asleep. In a study conducted by University of Pittsburgh sleep researcher Timothy Monk, for example, people were asked to report when they *felt* sleepy, what we might call *subjective sleepiness*. At the same time, they were given various chances throughout the day to actual- ly try to fall asleep.

When asked to report their sense of themselves around the middle of the day, most people said they felt wide awake. Yet tests showed that this was one of the sleepiest times of most people's day. That is, when given the chance to sleep, people fell asleep faster at this time than at any other daylight hour. In this instance, at least, subjective sleepiness and objective sleepiness were at odds.

Of course, it makes sense that we'd need *two* systems to control sleepiness and wakefulness. If our sleep-wake cy- cles operated inexorably on a fixed, twenty-four-hour sched- ule, we'd always fall asleep at the same time each night, no matter what the circumstances. Humans—and most other creatures—need to be more adaptable than that, more re- sponsive to actual changing conditions. So our sleep-wake cy- cle's own logic is to run free—to move ahead one hour each night, to expand into fifty-hour days—while our temperature cycle is more regular. Developing a regular sleep schedule al- lows us to associate our temperature cycles more closely with our sleep-wake cycles, while leaving us free to stay up late for any emergency that might come along.

Making Your Cycles Work for You

I always went to bed at least for one hour as early as possible in the afternoon and exploited to the full my happy gift of falling almost immediately to sleep. By this means I was able to press a day and a half's work into one. Nature had not intended mankind to work from eight in the morning until mid-night without the refreshment of blessed oblivion, which, even if it lasts only twenty minutes, is sufficient to renew all vital forces.

— Winston Churchill, *The Gathering Storm*

The more you know about your own bodily rhythms, the more you can work with them, rather than against them, to get the kind of sleep that's best for you. For example, for some of us naps are the solution to sleepless nights. For others, naps only make the problem worse. For still others, naps are a good solution—but only under certain circumstances.

How do you know which approach is right for you? The answer depends on knowing still more about sleep-wake cycles and temperature cycles.

Let's begin with a statistical observation: there seem to be two two-hour "troughs" when most humans are at their lowest and/or at their sleepiest. One low period is during the day—extending roughly from 2 to 4 P.M.—and the other is at night— extending roughly from 4 to 6 A.M. These troughs are indicated by such figures as the number of sleep-related auto accidents, deaths from illness and disease, industrial accidents, and the like.

There also seem to be some particularly wakeful times for most people. According to a number of studies, it's virtually impossible for most people to fall asleep during the hours of 7 to 10 P.M. On the other hand, it's extremely difficult for most people to wake up between 3 and 6 A.M.

Researchers believe that these wakeful and sleepy times are only the most intense of the many ultradian ups and downs that occur throughout our days and nights. Remember how sleep cycles seem to occur in ninety-minute periods—the time it takes to pass through four stages of sleep and a REM phase? (For more on sleep patterns, see Chapter 2.) Well, wakefulness cycles also occur in ninety-minute segments.

Of course, psychological and physical factors can affect any of these rhythms. Think of all the things that can speed up your breathing and slow it down. Then think of all the physical and psychological factors that can affect your ninety-minute cycles of sleepiness and wakefulness. Certainly, if you're attending an important meeting, a long-awaited romantic encounter, or an incredibly slow and boring movie, your "natural cycle" will be tempted to give way to the pressure of events.

Most of the time, our responsiveness to outside cues may not be a problem. However, if you're concerned about not getting enough sleep or about not feeling alert enough during the day, it may be to your advantage to rediscover your own inner rhythms and enlist them in your search for better sleep.

Here's where knowing whether you're a night owl or a lark can come in handy. Studies have shown that night owls seem to have markedly different temperature rhythms than larks. For example, sleep researcher Kaneyoshi Ishihara and his colleagues from four Japanese universities studied some fifteen hundred university students. Not only did larks go to bed and get up earlier than owls, but they seemed to fall asleep more easily and to feel more rested and more cheerful when they woke up.

Larks and night owls also differed in the way they took or didn't take naps. Whereas larks seemed more likely to feel they had gotten enough sleep at night, owls seemed to take longer and more frequent naps. Owls also took their naps later in the day than larks did, further suggesting that their temperature cycles were running on a later clock.

American studies seemed to confirm that owls are just not as good sleepers as larks. The Japanese researchers took issue with that value judgment, however, suggesting that owls were simply more flexible and irregular in their sleep habits. They found, for example, that owls' bedtimes and wake times could vary by as much as an hour or more, whereas larks' variation times usually stayed within half an hour or less. On weekends and holidays, owls were likely to stay up and sleep even later—delaying their rest by two to three hours—whereas larks tended to keep delays under two hours and were less likely to delay in the first place.

In our standardized society, such flexibility might lead to insufficient sleep. Since staying up later can't always be matched by sleeping later, the free-running owl will naturally have less of a chance to make up his or her lost sleep than the more regular lark. Hence, perhaps, their greater tendency to take naps, as well as their more frequent complaints about feeling sleepy.

Many night owls enjoy the fun and the freedom of staying up late, paying willingly for their pleasure with the price of less sleep. If this trade-off isn't working for you, however, you might consider trying for a more regular schedule, even if not an earlier one.

On the other hand, the Japanese studies showed that night owls' late hours did seem to have an internal logic. When they took EEG and body-temperature readings of ten larks and eleven owls (an admittedly small sample), they found that the larks' average late-night low point was 4:17 A.M., whereas the owls' trough came at 6:10 A.M.

Temperature differences between different sleep types were also noted by James Horne of England's Loughborough University and O. Östberg of the Swedish National Board of Occupational Safety and Health. The two researchers found that larks' body temperature tended to be higher than owls' throughout the day, and that larks' temperature tended to peak around 7:30 P.M. (the period of their greatest wakefulness), as opposed to 10:30 P.M. for owls. Then, after their respective peaks, larks' temperatures fell lower.

People who fell into neither the lark nor the night owl category in Horne and Östberg's study—"intermediate" types—had temperatures that fell between those of the other two. They alone of the three groups had a midafternoon trough that occurred betwen 3 and 6 P.M.

When it came to sleep times, the intermediate types in this study went to sleep with the larks, at about 11:30 P.M.—even though their evening temperatures peaked with the owls', at about 10:30 P.M. (That's still more evidence that our sleep-wake cycles and our temperature cycles aren't always in synch.) The owls, of course, didn't go to bed until about 1 A.M. Yet all three groups slept from eight to eight and a half hours. Studies from France, Italy, the Netherlands, and the United States have confirmed these patterns.

Interestingly, although the larks in the Japanese study reported feeling better upon arising, EEG measurements showed no objective differences in sleep quality between the two groups. In other words, just because you get up grouchy at 10 A.M. and your mate wakes up singing at seven, your mate's sleep wasn't necessarily any better than your own. You may just have different subjective experiences of waking up.

You may also be interested to know that larks and owls didn't differ significantly on personality tests, although there was a slight tendency for owls to be more extroverted, nervous, and anxious. It's hard to know whether that reflects a true personality difference—or simply the fallout from living in a society in which early risers are considered more hardworking and reliable than late sleepers.

How might all this knowledge affect your decisions about whether, when, and how to take naps? Well, like much else in sleep research, naps are a controversial topic. Some experts recommend naps for poor sleepers and/or insomniacs, seeing them as a way to respond to our natural tendency to have two troughs during the twenty-four-hour day. Particularly if you can time your nap so that you are sleeping during your "low time," these experts would see a nap as a practical and refreshing solution.

Other experts see naps as interfering with the insomniac's ability to get a good *night's* sleep. It's certainly true that if your sleep and wake times are irregular, and particularly if you're going to bed later and later each night, a daily nap can interfere with your ability to regularize your sleep.

Some specialists say that naps aren't good for insomniacs who wake up too early—particularly if they're waking up after 6 A.M. They say that the insomniac who can't fall asleep at night may want to avoid naps, at least while he or she is trying to regularize a sleep schedule.

On the other hand, the notion that an afternoon nap will inevitably keep you from falling asleep at night is not true for everyone. Dr. Philip Tiller conducted an experiment at the Louisiana State School of Medicine. He encouraged several hundred women who had complained of nervous fatigue to take a one-or two-hour nap every afternoon— and found that this actually helped them sleep *better* at night, as well as improving the other symptoms of two-thirds of the women.

If you do nap, how long should your sleep be? Again, no one has an answer that applies to everyone. You're unlikely to get much REM sleep in an afternoon nap that's less than two hours (unless you're in REM rebound)—but the benefit of an afternoon nap may be in its ability to provide deep non-REM sleep. According to Dr. Timothy Roehrs of the Henry Ford Hospital in Detroit, the amount of deep sleep in afternoon naps is unusually high.

Dr. Charles Fisher, a New York psychoanalyst who has spent the last twenty-five years researching sleep, points out that many people seem to benefit from extremely short naps. He says, "We still don't know, scientifically, why so short a sleep—ten minutes, one minute—can be refreshing to many people. It could be that it stops conscious thought processes, and in this way relieves anxiety. Or, as has been found, non-dreaming sleep helps the problem-solving mechanism."

Sleep studies have shown that we tend to feel sleepy and alert at the same times each day, regardless of the total amount of sleep we've gotten the night or the week before. That is, even if you've stayed up all night, you'll feel much the same ups and downs that you'd have felt anyway. Even in sleep-deprivation experiments, in which subjects are allowed virtually no sleep for several days at a time, people report feeling alert and sleepy according to their regular rhythms, however much of an overall "downward pull" their sleep deprivation may exert.

From that point of view, it may be more helpful to think of naps not in relation to getting an abstract total amount of sleep, but as a way to swing with your own daily rhythms. Picture your entire twenty-four-hour day and begin to ask yourself when you feel alert, and when you feel sleepy; when you'd like to be awake, and when you'd prefer to be asleep. Once you've discovered your own internal rhythms, you can decide whether and how naps fit into them.

Dancing to Your Own Rhythms

We are not meant to fight against nature's waves; we are meant to ride with them, and our bodies experience a need to do that. It's only when we interfere with the process that we experience discomfort, whether from insomnia or anything else.

— Deepak Chopra

You might imagine charting your rhythms as a number of concentric circles. At the center are the shortest, most oft-repeated rhythms—your heartbeat, the blinking of your eyes, the time it takes you to breathe in and out. Surrounding these tiny rhythms are the ninety-minute cycles of sleep and wakefulness. The next circle charts the pattern of your day, with one big sleepy period in the afternoon and another, bigger sleepy period at night. Finally, you can see your largest rhythms—such as your menstrual cycle and your responsiveness to the changing seasons.

As your awareness grows, you should find it progressively easier to imagine ways of arranging your schedule so that you can work with, rather than against, your own rhythms. If you realize you're a "late person," for example, do you have the option of arranging a later starting time for your job, if you agree to stay later and/or to take work home? If you're an early riser, can you come in to work an hour earlier and take the extra time in the form of a midday nap? At the very least, you may be able to schedule your most important meetings or challenging projects during the times of day or evening that you've discovered you're most alert. Working in tune with your own rhythms can have a profound effect on your insomnia, simply by making you feel more relaxed and more responsive to your body.

If you must accommodate to a work schedule that seems foreign to your nature, take heart. Most people can learn to adapt to any schedule if they give themselves a month to get used to it and stick with enormous discipline to regular sleep and wake times. Willy-nilly, this happens to many night owls when they have children. If their children are early risers, the parents *will* rise early in the morning. Children are probably the most powerful environmental reinforcement of all.

Even if you don't have children, you can develop a regular sleep-wake schedule, but you may need outside reinforcement to do so. You might need to enlist a sleeping partner, roommate, friend, or temporary live-in relative, as the process may take about a month. Some people need the reinforcement of checking into a hospital to "reset their clocks," primarily such independent types as freelance workers who live alone and as such have no ongoing reasons to conform to a daily routine.

The easiest way to regularize your schedule is to pick a bedtime and wake time and stick to it. Avoid naps if you have difficulty falling asleep, and *make sure you get up when you say you will*, no matter when you went to bed. Within a month, you should be functioning normally.

If that doesn't work for you, you might try going around the clock. Simply go to bed and get up two hours later each day. Eventually, you'll have brought your clock around to an early bedtime—say, 11 P.M.—paired with a correspondingly early wake time. You need to commit a week to ten days to delay your clock in this way, however, as in the middle of the process you'll be sleeping during the day.

Some people work backward, advancing their bedtimes and wake times. This works for some early risers, to help them sleep later, but most people find it too hard to go to bed earlier rather than later.

Another rhythmic influence on our sleep is the amount of sunlight available during the day. The so-called seasonal affective disorder (SAD) has been known to cause depression, sleep disorders, and other symptoms in certain people who seem particularly sensitive to reduced light during the winter. Exposure to bright light has been used to treat these people with some success.

Most sleep researchers don't believe that any time of day is a priori better or worse for sleeping. On the contrary, all research seems to indicate that humans are remarkably flexible in what they're able to adapt to—even if this adaptation sometimes comes at a cost. If you can find your own comfortable rhythms, and set up a support system to reinforce them, you may be surprised at how much more easily and deeply you find yourself sleeping.

Chapter 6

Natural Sleep Remedies

*Gradually, he fell into that deep tranquil sleep
which ease from recent suffering alone imparts; that
calm and peaceful rest which it is pain to wake
from. Who, if this were death, would be roused
again to all the struggles and turmoils of life; to all
its cares for the present; its anxieties for the future;
more than all, its weary recollections of the past!*

—Dickens, *Oliver Twist*

No matter how troubled our sleep may often be, each of us has a memory of at least one time when that "deep tranquil sleep" described by Dickens belonged to us, as well. In this chapter, you'll find a number of suggestions for how to re-create that sleep.

Dickens, by the way, often suffered from insomnia himself, which may be why he wrote so frequently and feelingly about sleep. As he put it in his first novel, *The Pickwick Papers*, "Every one has experienced that disagreeable state of mind, in which a sensation of bodily weariness contends against an inability to sleep."

Certainly, prescription and over-the-counter sleep aids were not unknown in Dickens' time. Laudanum, opium, and other sedatives made frequent appearances in many a Victorian novel. Dickens himself, though, favored more natural remedies. When Mr. Pickwick "came to the conclusion that it was of no use trying to sleep . . . he got up and . . . dressed himself." Dickens waxed more autobiographical in "Night Walks," an essay that appeared in *The Uncommercial Traveller*:

> . . . a temporary inability to sleep, referable to a distressing impression, caused me to walk about the streets all night. The disorder might have taken a long time to conquer, if it had been faintly experimented on in bed, but it was soon defeated by the brisk treatment of getting up directly after lying down, and going out, and coming home tired at sunrise. . . . My last special feat was turning out of bed at two . . . and walking thirty miles into the country to breakfast . . . fell asleep to the monotonous sound of my own feet, doing their regular four miles an hour . . . dozing heavily and dreaming constantly . . .

In this chapter, you'll find suggestions for sleep-inducing aerobic exercise remarkably similar to Dickens's self-prescription. You'll also find descriptions of a number of other natural sleep remedies: relaxation techniques, meditation, sensory healing techniques, massage, and biofeedback.

Finally, this chapter introduces alternative healing traditions: chiropractic, the Chinese medical tradition of acupuncture and herbal remedies, and the Ayurvedic medical tradition of India. What these traditions have in common is a holistic approach to mind, body, and spirit—an approach that is singularly well suited to what Western medicine would term "psychophysiological insomnia," in which physical and psychological causes are intertwined.

It can be freeing to remember how interrelated these three dimensions are, to realize that a positive change in any one dimension may bring about unlooked-for benefits in the other two. Virtually every technique suggested in this chapter has the potential for resonating throughout your life in unexpected ways. Use your intuition to choose which suggestions you'd like to experiment with and in what order.

First, though, a word about sleeping pills.

Sleeping Pills, Tranquilizers, and Other Drugs

> Not poppy, nor mandragora,
> Nor all the drowsy syrups of the world,
> Shall ever medicine thee to that sweet sleep,
> Which thou owedst yesterday.
> —Shakespeare, *Othello*

You may be surprised to discover that sleeping pills actually militate against good, deep, refreshing sleep. Whereas the other remedies described in this chapter all have beneficial side effects, sleeping pills' *only* good effect is to enable you to lose consciousness on a night when you might otherwise not be able to. Some nights, this may be such a desirable goal that taking a pill is completely worth it to you. But for a long-term solution to your sleep problems, pills are probably not the answer.

The use of sleeping pills in the United States probably peaked in the 1970s, when many new medications came onto the market and the dangers of using sleep aids were not yet well known. In those days, doctors wrote nearly 40 million prescriptions for sleep aids a year. Even today, some 8 million people still take prescription sleeping pills, and another 20-to-22 million take over-the-counter sleep medications. Only aspirin sales are higher. One researcher estimated U.S. residents take enough sleeping medication to put every man, woman, and child in the country to sleep for two hundred hours!

According to psychiatrists Stuart Yudofsky and Robert E. Hales and physician Tom Ferguson, authors of *What You Need to Know About Psychiatric Drugs*, 30 percent of all sleeping pill prescriptions are written for people whose primary problem is psychiatric (that is, depression, or some other psychiatric condition is producing their insomnia); 25 percent are written for people with medical problems (that is, their insomnia is secondary to some physical problem, such as ulcers, that is interfering with their sleep); and 18 percent are written for people with ill-defined or vague symptoms (that is, the doctors aren't sure what the problem is, but it includes difficulty sleeping). Only about 15 percent of sleep medication prescriptions are written for people whose primary problem is simply that they can't sleep.

Many doctors prescribe sleeping pills as a kind of automatic first response to hearing about or anticipating a sleep problem. About 50 percent of all hospital patients are routinely prescribed sleeping pills—and 20 percent of those will later become dependent on their medication. Moreover, some 50 percent of those who take sleeping pills to treat their insomnia develop even *worse* sleeping problems than they had when they started.

What can a sleeping pill accomplish? Typically, for someone with insomnia, it can speed the onset of sleep by some five to twenty minutes. Medication does tend to cut down on the number of times an insomniac will wake up during the night, and it will probably extend total sleep time. In the long run, however, if you rely on sleeping pills to help you sleep, you'll probably end up sleeping less and feeling even more frustrated with your inability to achieve restful sleep.

A sleeping pill may be effective for three to seven nights. If a person needs to recover from a major trauma—the death of a loved one, a major move, the stressful beginning of a new job—sleeping medication may be appropriate for this short time, to help people under extreme stress avoid the emotional consequences of a sleepless night. After that, sleeping pills lose their effectiveness anyway. According to Drs. Yudofsky, Hales, and Ferguson, a person who takes sleep medication for more than a week takes just as long to fall asleep, wakes just as often, and sleeps for no more total time than a person with the same problem who takes no medication. Moreover, a person who takes sleeping pills regularly faces a 50 percent higher risk of accidental death.

Sleep medications stay in your body far longer than the time it takes you to fall asleep and wake up. That's why people who have kidney or liver disease, or who are over sixty-five, should not take sleep medications in any case. Sleep medication must be metabolized by the liver (which, as we saw, experiences it as a toxin) and is eventually excreted by the kidneys, so if either organ is functioning improperly, the medication can remain in your body for even longer than otherwise. Likewise, if you're over sixty-five, your body takes longer to metabolize and excrete medication, so sleep medication will also remain in your body for far too long.

Of course, no one should combine sleep medication with alcohol, or take sleep medication while pregnant. Nor should anyone with respiratory problems take sleep medication, as it can interfere with the brain's ability to regulate breathing.

Even if you don't fit into any of these categories, you risk the following side effects, from either prescription or over-the-counter sleep aids:

❭ Fatal overdose, especially when combined with alcohol or with other drugs that affect your central nervous system

❭ Impaired coordination, memory, driving skills, and thinking

❭ Interference with breathing

❭ Physical or psychological dependence—i.e., you become unable to sleep *without* the medication

❭ Tolerance—i.e., you need to take larger and larger doses to achieve the same effect

❭ Potential damage to kidney, liver, and lungs

❭ Confusion, hallucinations, and similar disturbances, particularly for the elderly

The most commonly prescribed medications for sleep are the benzodiazepines, a group of antianxiety drugs that includes flurazepam (Dalmane), temazepam (Restoril), and triazolam (Halcion), as well as other drugs in this family that are generally not prescribed to treat sleep problems although they may help induce sleep—e.g., alprazolam (Xanax), diazepam (Valium), chlordiazepoxide (Librium), and several others.

The mechanisms by which benzodiazepines produce their effects is not completely understood, but it seems to have something to do with affecting the brain's neurotransmitters, those biochemicals that help neurons (nerve cells) communicate. (For more on the biology of sleep, see Chapter

2.) Flurazepam, temazepam, and triazolam all reduce body movements and total night awakenings while lowering the number of shifts from one sleep stage to another. However, they also suppress REM sleep and decrease the deep sleep that comes in Stages 3 and 4.

All benzodiazepines pose a high risk for physical and psychological dependence. Stopping these medications after some weeks of use can also produce painful withdrawal symptoms—severe anxiety, nervous agitation, and the inability to sleep. All discontinuance of benzodiazepines should be carried out gradually and under a doctor's care.

Even if you've only taken these medications for a week or more, you may develop *rebound insomnia*—a difficulty sleeping *without* the drug once you've grown used to sleeping *with* the drug. If you feel you're developing such a syndrome, don't start taking the drug again. Instead, work with a physician to find another solution.

The other major category of prescription sleeping pills is known as *barbiturates*. These are classified according to how long they remain active within the body. It's the intermediate-acting barbiturates that are used as sleeping pills, including amobarbital (Amytal), pentobarbital (Nembutal), and secobarbital (Seconal). Basically, barbiturates depress the central nervous system, interfering with the passage of impulses within the brain. In other words, they knock you out. Rather than inducing sleep—which, as we've seen, is a complicated physiological process—they just disrupt the chemical processes of the brain so that you're unable to function consciously.

Like benzodiazepines, barbiturates interfere with the deep sleep of Stages 3 and 4, as well as suppressing REM sleep. Like other sleep aids, they are highly addictive, interfere with coordination and other key functions, and may be fatal when combined with alcohol.

Perhaps the best distinction between natural sleep and narcosis (drug-induced unconsciousness) comes from Dr. Herbert Sheldon, who says:

> Drugs do not produce sleep. . . . In sleep the body is normally engaged in its most efficient reparative and building processes; in narcosis it is engaged in resisting and throwing off poison. This is the reason that sleep is a process of renewal and recuperation, while narcosis is an exhaustive process. The first conserves energy, the second wastes energy. Following sleep, the muscles are stronger; following narcosis the muscles are weak and tremulous. The will is weakened by narcosis; it is strengthened by sleep.

If you still feel that sleeping medications are useful for you in some circumstances, here are some suggestions:

❭ Avoid over-the-counter medications altogether. Don't ever use medication prescribed for a friend. Instead, get a prescription from your physician—preferably one who's quite familiar with your entire medical history as well as with your personality and relationship to medication. That way, if you begin to develop side effects, dependence, or other difficulty, you'll have a partner to help you work through the problems. Over-the-counter medication is also less effective than prescription pills while being at least as hazardous.

❭ Never refill a prescription for sleep aids without your doctor's explicit awareness.

❭ Discuss all side effects, rebound effects, and potential dependency with your doctor at the time the medication is prescribed.

❭ If your doctor seems too casual in writing a sleep-aid prescription, you might want to get a second opinion.

❭ Learn more about sleep medication by reading *What You Need to Know About Psychiatric Drugs* or *Drug Information for the Consumer* by Consumer Reports Books.

❭ Don't take medication on the same night your sleeping partner does, so that one of you will be alert to deal with a nighttime emergency.

❭ Avoid medication on the night before a long drive or strenuous activity— the chemicals will remain in your system the next day and may continue to cause drowsiness.

❭ Never combine sleep medication with liquor or any other medication that affects the central nervous system.

❭ Never give any type of sleep aid to children.

Nature's Remedies

The wise man thinks about his troubles only when there is some purpose in doing so; at other times he thinks about other things, or, if at night, about nothing at all.

—Bertrand Russell

How can you get to that blessed state of thinking about "nothing at all" at night? There are a number of routes to this goal, any or all of which might be right for you.

Vigorous exercise during the day and mild exercise at bedtime will not only help you fall asleep and stay asleep more easily but will increase the amount of time you spend in deepest Stage 4 sleep. Just about everyone seems to feel better when exercise becomes a part of his or her daily routine, and some people overcome their sleep problems through exercise alone. After all, your body was meant to be used.

Exercise seems to reduce stress by helping to dissipate the lactic acid that accumulates in the blood. It also eases the muscular tension that can build up, sharpens the brain by increasing the amount of oxygen that travels there, strengthens and stimulates the heart and lungs, vitalizes the nervous system, activates the endocrine system, and increases the body's production of endorphins, a natural morphinelike product that creates a sense of well-being and increases the body's resistance to pain. Exercise also stimulates the release of epinephrine, a hormone that likewise creates a sense of happiness and excitement. People who exercise regularly report feeling far less boredom, worry, and tension.

To help combat sleeplessness, it's best to get some form of aerobic exercise—exercise that increases the amount of oxygen that reaches the blood. Aerobic exercise includes, for example, jogging, swimming, riding a bicycle, jumping rope, dancing, riding a stationary bicycle, using a treadmill, and walking. Weightlifting is not usually aerobic exercise, although it may have other benefits.

Whatever exercise you choose, make sure it involves vigorous use of your legs. According to Dr. Paul Dudley White, "The fatigue produced by [using leg muscles] is undoubtedly the best tranquilizer ever made, either by nature or man."

You don't need to become a top athlete for exercise to make you feel better. And you don't need to devote enormous amounts of time to it. A mild workout for fifteen to twenty minutes a day, four days a week, will be enough for you to feel the benefits. Be sure, though, to stretch before and after you do anything vigorous, and to allow yourself a cool-down period after exercising, before you stretch.

For many people, the ideal time to exercise is early in the morning, when the air is still fresh and when the lift in body temperature helps them wake up. If your main concern is combating insomnia, you may have better luck exercising at the end of the afternoon or in the early evening: you'll be more tired at bedtime, and you'll have more chance of dissipating the day's mental and physical tensions. In any case, avoid vigorous late-night exercise, since, as you'll notice, exercise helps you wake up.

If you feel tense and keyed-up at the end of an evening, some mild, non-aerobic exercise may do you good. A leisurely walk in which you breathe deeply and allow yourself to respond to the physical sensation of being outside could be helpful. Gentle dancing to pleasant music can also help you lift your mood and relax your body. Yoga and stretching exercises can also be good ways to wind down.

Exercise itself is relaxing, but you may also want to focus more specifically on relaxation to help you sleep. The most commonly recommended relaxation technique is *progressive relaxation*, invented in the 1940s by Dr. Edmund Jacobson of the Laboratory for Clinical Psychology.

The key to progressive relaxation is to become aware of tension and its corresponding state, relaxation, in each of the body's muscles. If you can commit from fifteen minutes to an hour a day for a week to ten days, you can teach yourself how to relax completely, at will. Then you can induce a state of relaxation that will carry you into slumber.

The following exercise is meant to be done in a quiet room—not necessarily dark—on a comfortable bed, couch, or exercise pad. You might want to record the following four paragraphs on a tape to listen to as you relax, or have a friend make the recording. Be sure to pause often enough to give yourself time to relax.

Lie down and get comfortable. Allow your spine to sink into the bed. Feel your weight pulling you down. Find a comfortable position for your arms and legs. Allow your eyes to close. Feel your breath moving in and out, filling your body, traveling to each muscle. Don't push your breathing, allow your breath to travel through your body. You don't have to do any work—your breath just happens. Feel it moving in and out. Feel your spine sinking comfortably into the bed. Allow yourself to relax.

Very gradually, allow yourself to stiffen your arms, slowly. Do not clench your fists. Do not move your arms. Allow your arms to remain still and your hands to remain open. Stiffen your arm muscles so that they're just a little tight. Hold them there for a count of ten. One, two, three, four . . . Now stiffen them a little bit more, and hold for another count of ten. One, two, three, four . . . Now stiffen them still more. Hold for a count of thirty. One, two, three, four . . .

How do your arms feel? Can you feel how dull and tight your muscles are? When have you felt this way before? Let your mind travel into your arms. Feel everything you can about this state of tension. How does your skin feel? How do your shoulders feel? What do you notice about your elbows, fore-arms, wrists, fingers? Allow yourself to notice every-thing about your arms.

Now relax your arms slowly, a little at a time. What do you notice about that taut, tense feeling? Continue to relax your arms. Feel how your arm mus-cles are loose and warm. Feel the blood circulating through your arm muscles, through your shoulders, upper arms, elbows, forearms, wrists, fingers. Feel how the blood warms your arms. How does the skin feel? How do the muscles feel? Allow your breath to travel through your arm muscles, relaxing them fur-ther, letting them fall loosely by your sides. Feel their weight as they relax. What else do you notice? Continue to allow your arms to relax and allow your-self to enjoy the feeling.

You might repeat this exercise two more times, for a total of about forty-five minutes of relaxation time. When you feel you've learned how to relax your arms, you can repeat the procedure with other muscles—legs, chest, abdomen, and face. Each time, you begin by tensing the muscles, holding the tension, and then relaxing.

Eventually, you'll be able to go straight to the relax-ation mode, and when you're lying in bed, awake, you'll be able to identify where you're tense and allow yourself to relax. However, if you're ever having trouble sleeping, it's always a good idea to make tense muscles *more* tense before relaxing them. You may feel that relaxing your muscles is out of your control, but you can *always* make a muscle more tense. Doing so reminds you that in fact, they're your muscles, so you can relax them if you want to.

Many people find it helpful to check in with themselves and their muscles throughout the day. Asking yourself where you notice tension—face? lower back? legs?—and allowing yourself to breathe and relax will help you end your entire day in a more relaxed state.

The relaxation technique described above is presented as a learning technique, but you can use it—with some variation—as you're trying to fall asleep. You might make a tape of it, or just learn how to say these words silently to yourself.

When you're trying to become completely relaxed, always begin by getting comfortable and breathing deeply. Always think of breath as moving in and out of your body by itself, as a process that you're allowing to happen rather than as one you're forcing or pushing. Many people find it helpful to progressively relax head, face, chin, neck, shoulders, spine, lower back, chest, arms, elbows, hands, fingers, abdomen, hips, groin, thighs, knees, calves, ankles, and toes. If you're making a tape, include instructions for all these body parts, allowing plenty of time to return to your breathing in between each one. You might also include an instruction like the following: "If you notice tension anywhere, allow yourself to feel it and let it go"; or "If any muscle anywhere is tense, tighten it further and then release it."

Another relaxation option is to focus on the eyes and the face muscles. According to Dr. Jacobson, "If eyes and speech organs are really relaxed (as measured electronically) for even as short a time as thirty seconds, the person is asleep at the end of this time."

Here are two techniques that you can use to relax your eyes and face muscles. Again, you can make a tape or learn to say your own version of these instructions silently to yourself. You can practice either or both exercises at a time of day when you're *not* trying to sleep, so you have time to learn the techniques before you try to use them:

1. Lie down and allow yourself to get comfortable. Breathe deeply. Feel the breath moving in and out. Close your eyes.

Tightly wrinkle your forehead by raising your eyebrows as high as they will go. Hold them up for a minute or so. Count to sixty as you hold them: one, two, three. . . As you count, explore the feeling of tension in your forehead. Can you feel each of your muscles? Where does each muscle begin? Where does it end? How does the skin of your forehead feel when the muscles are tense? Is it hot or cool? Can you feel the blood running throughout your forehead? What else do you notice?

Now, gradually, let your forehead relax. Allow your forehead to relax for five minutes. What do you notice? Does it feel hot or cool? Can you feel the breath reaching the muscles in your forehead. Where does each muscle begin and end now? Can you feel how loose your relaxed muscles are? Can you feel how heavy they are? What else do you notice?

Next, close your eyelids tightly. Hold them that way for thirty seconds: one, two, three . . .

Notice everything you can about your tightly closed eyelids. Then allow them to relax. (Again, you can repeat two or three times if necessary.)

2. Lie down. Get comfortable. Allow yourself to breathe deeply. Feel the breath move in and out.

Close your eyelids tightly. Without moving your head, allow the eyes to roll upward so that you're "looking up." Hold this position for thirty seconds: one, two, three . . . What do you notice about the tension in your eyes? Allow yourself to keep noticing.

Now relax your eyes, completely. Let them lie straight in their sockets. What do you notice? Allow your eyes to stay relaxed for five minutes. Keep noticing. Keep breathing deeply.

Now allow your eyes to roll so that you're "looking down" without moving your head. What do you notice? Hold this position for thirty seconds: one, two, three . . .

Once again, relax, breathe, and notice. Now look left without moving your head. What do you notice? Hold this position for thirty seconds: one, two, three . . . Once again, relax, breathe, and notice.

Now allow yourself to look right without moving your head. What do you notice? Hold this position for thirty seconds: one, two, three . . . Continue to breathe. Finally, relax again.

Although people who meditate say they find it relaxing, meditation involves your mind and body in far different ways than progressive relaxation. According to psychologist

Donald E. Miskiman of the University of Alberta, "Transcendental Meditation [one form of meditation] seems to stabilize the sleep-dream cycle by reducing the effect of any disruption to this cycle and thereby restoring the system more quickly to its normal level of functioning." Miskiman studied insomniacs who averaged 75.6 minutes of waking time before they finally fell asleep; thirty days after learning to meditate, they were falling asleep in 15.1 minutes—a perfectly normal time.

Those who have meditated for several months note that, as time goes by, the sleep they get is deeper and more refreshing, and they generally note feeling more alert and relaxed throughout the day.

If you're interested in learning to meditate, remember to give it time. Although some people experience quick, dramatic improvements in their insomnia, for others it takes longer. A peaceful, accepting attitude will help you get the most out of your meditation.

Meditation can't be taught in a book; you'll have to find a private instructor or a class. Look in the yellow pages under "Transcendental Meditation" (this form of meditation is supported by an international organization), or ask at your local health-food store. You might also look up "Yoga" in the phone book, as any place that teaches yoga may either teach meditation or be able to recommend someone who does.

Did you ever think of the biochemical effect of using your senses? Everything we see, hear, touch, smell, or taste affects the chemistry of our brain as we take in and process the perception. For that reason, Ayurvedic and Western doctor Deepak Chopra suggests using soothing sensory stimulation to help ease your senses to sleep. He points to studies that showed hospital patients improving more quickly when they had a pleasing view to look at, and advises troubled sleepers to decorate their bedrooms in gentle colors and with beautiful objects.

Music can likewise comfort the senses, both during the day and at bedtime. Chopra particularly recommends Gandharva-veda music, which has been specially composed for healing in the Ayurvedic tradition.

To heal through the skin, Chopra suggests massage. Before your morning or evening bath, try a sesame oil massage for the body, or just for the bottoms of the feet; particularly intense people might try coconut oil instead.

Healing smells include warm, sweet, and sour scents: basil, orange, rose, geranium, cloves, and other spices. The smells can be burned as incense or oils or enjoyed in bath oils. Oil of lavender rubbed on the forehead may also be therapeutic.

Biofeedback is a scientifically sophisticated way to learn the relaxation that you may have practiced on your own through relaxation exercises. Basically, biofeedback consists of being hooked up to a machine that measures certain *biological* reactions—including body temperature, muscle relaxation, and breathing rate—and gives you *feedback* about them, in the form of a sounding buzzer, a flashing light, or the biofeedback therapist's reaction as he or she reads your printout. Apparently, by getting feedback on apparently involuntary processes, human beings learn to control these processes at will.

If you're interested in learning more about biofeedback, ask your physician for a referral, as it can only be done under laboratory conditions with trained technicians. For many people, particularly those who are resistant to relaxation exercises, meditation, and other individual forms of treatment, the partnership with the therapist proves very effective.

Alternative Healing

> Sleep, that knits up the ravell'd sleave of care,
> The death of each day's life, sore labour's bath,
> Balm of hurt minds, great nature's second course,
> Chief nourisher in life's feast.
>
> —Shakespeare, *Macbeth*

Alternative systems of healing have become quite controversial in recent years. Growing numbers of middle-class, middle-aged, and otherwise "respectable" people have begun to experiment with healing techniques that were once considered the sole province of New Age fanatics. Many insurance companies will now reimburse members for chiropractic and even acupuncture. Asian medicine has also won a new prestige and respectability in the West.

Many Western-trained doctors view this phenomenon with alarm. They point out that there is little regulation of alternative healers, that many of their claims have no basis in scientific fact, and that as long as patients are seduced into believing that their conditions are receiving alternate treatment, they will fail to get proper medical care from trained physicians.

If your insomnia has appeared with any other troubling symptoms, or if you have any suspicion that it may be related to a more serious illness, you should certainly reassure yourself by getting a thorough checkup from a trained medical physician or sleep specialist physician. However, it's also true that Western medicine's specialty is more in the realm of dramatic interventions. Treating daily, chronic, nonlife-threatening conditions—insomnia, backache, fatigue, and low spirits—is simply not what most Western doctors have been trained to do.

Alternative medical traditions, on the other hand, while less effective in dealing with a difficult birth, a failing heart, or a sudden emergency, are often more effective in addressing what we might call issues of "wellness." In other words, if your health is basically good but you have trouble sleeping, an alternative medical tradition may have a lot to offer you, particularly if you maintain close contact with your Western practitioner.

You should make very sure, however, that you are dealing with a healer who is licensed and credentialed within his or her own tradition. Unless you've been referred to your practitioner by someone you trust implicitly, it's appropriate to ask the alternative healer to describe his or her credentials and even to give references. At the very least, the practitioner should describe clearly what treatment you'll receive, what results you can expect from it, how long it's likely to take, and what it should cost.

As with any physician, you'll want to approach an alternative practitioner in a cooperative and open spirit—while at the same time allowing yourself to ask questions, express doubts, and share in the responsibility for your own treatment. And, as with any physician, in the end, your own intuition is probably your strongest guide as to what works for you.

If you'd like to explore alternative medicine but aren't sure where to start, you might check the bulletin boards or ask the counter person at your local health-food store or restaurant. The bulletin boards at dance studios often list chiropractors and similar alternative professionals. "Acupuncture" may be listed in the yellow pages or business white pages of your local phone book, as might "Homeopathy."

Here is a brief description of each alternative discipline and how it works. For more detailed information, talk with a practitioner and with some of his or her patients, so that you can decide whether these healing techniques are for you.

Chiropractic is based on the principle that every organ connects to the spinal column, so that distress in an organ leads to a misalignment of the spine, and vice versa. Chiropractic adjustments of the spine are supposed to ease individual organs, back pains, and a host of other ailments as the body's entire sense of balance is restored. Chiropractors claim that adjustments of the spine help ease muscular problems, blood flow, and nervous disorders.

Some insomniacs have indeed claimed to be helped by occasional chiropractic adjustments.

Many chiropractors now offer counseling in nutrition and other forms of holistic medicine as well.

Ayurveda—Sanskrit for "the science of life"—is probably the oldest medical tradition in the world, dating as far back as 3000 B.C. according to some sources. In India, it's still a living tradition, and such popular figures as Deepak Chopra are helping to make it a treatment of interest in the United States and Europe.

Ayurvedic medicine focuses not on sickness but on wellness and balance. In this tradition, all of us are governed by three basic metabolic principles, or *doshas*: *vata*, which rules movement in the body; *pitta*, which rules energy, heat, and digestion; and *kapha*, the solid structure of the body. In each of us, a single dosha predominates, but all three must be in balance. The doshas govern all the rest of the universe as well, for Ayurveda is based on the principle that "the world is as we are." Thus, the hours of 6 P.M. to 10 P.M. are associated with kapha, and if you want to take advantage of slow, heavy kapha, you should be asleep by 10 P.M. Likewise, the hours of 2 A.M. to 6 A.M. are ruled by quick-moving vata, so waking before 6 A.M. is likely to cause agitation and distress.

Ayurvedic medicine also includes an elaborate system of diet (some indications of this have been given in Chapter 4), as well as a holistic approach to health involving meditation, purification practices, yogic exercises, care for the senses, and the like.

The *Chinese medical tradition* includes both acupuncture and herbal medicine. Acupuncture is based on the principle that the body consists of interconnected fields of energy. Acupuncture points are crucial junctures in those fields, which correspond to many parts and systems of the body simultaneously. Inserting acupuncture "needles"—which have the thickness of thread—at key acupuncture points helps to correct the energy flow of the body, restore vitality, right imbalances, and cure many disorders.

Acupuncture is particularly effective with those chronic, nonorganic (not attributable to a known physical agent) disorders that tend to baffle Western medicine, such as headache, fatigue, and of course, insomnia. Many people who go to acupuncturists for other ailments report immediate improvements in their sleeping habits, particularly the sensation of sleep that comes easily, lasts without interruption, and is deeper and more refreshing than they're used to.

Herbal medicine in the Chinese tradition is also based on the notion of restoring a balance. Yin—the passive, yielding, dark, and feminine aspects—must be in balance with yang—the dynamic, rational, active, light, and masculine aspects. An herbal healer will also see the body in terms of such elements as earth, air, fire, and water, and seek to restore these to balance as well.

Melatonin

In spite of recent enthusiastic publicity surrounding it, melatonin was little known until ten years ago, when research breakthroughs began to reveal some interesting and controversial findings related to this amazing substance. Some of its enthusiastic proponents maintain that melatonin is a wonder "drug" that can halt aging, battle cancer, boost the immune system, restore a vital sex drive, relieve stress, overcome jet lag, and cure insomnia.

Some advocates of melatonin also claim that it has an important role in combating, treating, or preventing AIDS, Alzheimer's disease, asthma, cataracts, diabetes, Down's syndrome and Parkinson's disease. They also believe that it can be the basis of a new estrogen-free birth-control pill that combats breast cancer at the same time that it prevents conception.

Melatonin and Sleep

Several studies suggest that melatonin may be a kind of "natural" sleeping pill, inducing sleep without suppressing REM (dream) sleep, as sedatives and other artificial sleep aids do. Travelers have started using melatonin to "reset their clocks" after flying across one or more time zones, and some studies seem to confirm melatonin's efficacy in combating jet lag and restoring restful sleep patterns.

How Does Melatonin Work?

To understand more about how melatonin produces its effects, we have to understand that it occurs naturally as a secretion of the pineal gland.

The pineal gland is a small organ behind the eyes that in reptiles is literally a "third eye"—a light-sensitive organ covered with a shield of clear cartilage. In humans, the pineal is hidden within the brain, although Hindu philosophy refers to a "third eye" that sees more deeply and truly than the other two. Indeed, the pineal does "see" in a way, for one of its jobs is to respond to changes in light and dark. Many living creatures possess a pineal gland, which some scientists now believe is a kind of natural clock, helping us to synchronize our activities with nature.

The pineal gland helps govern circadian rhythms— the biological rhythms that take place over a day, such as the sleep-wake cycle. This may be one of the reasons why it feels "natural" to sleep at night.

The pineal gland also governs seasonal rhythms that take place over weeks or months. By registering changes in the length of each day, for example, the pineal gland helps creatures know how the seasons are changing. Animals who mate in the spring are responding to hormonal changes set off by the pineal gland, as are animals who migrate in the fall or hibernate in the winter.

Women who menstruate every twenty eight days or so are also following a kind of seasonal rhythm, keeping time to the pineal clock. Indeed, researchers have noticed that women's pineal glands are larger than men's, perhaps because women need more internal time cues than men do, to help regulate their menstrual patterns. (Women's larger pineal glands may also help women live longer than men.)

Walter Pierpaoli, pioneer of much of the research into the function of the pineal gland, sees this organ as a kind of orchestra conductor. Just as an orchestra is comprised of a lot of different instruments, so is the human body made up of many different systems. The orchestra conductor tells each group of instruments when to start playing, how loudly to play, and when to stop; likewise, the pineal gland "tells" our endocrine and immune systems when and how to release key substances—growth hormones, sexual hormones, and antibodies.

How does the pineal gland "tell" other systems what to do? Pierpaoli believes that the messenger is melatonin. Changes in our levels of melatonin tell the body to enter puberty and begin sexual development. Melatonin may also be the trigger that sets the menstrual cycle in motion, that puts us to sleep, and that alerts our bodies to produce antibodies to combat disease. The complicated music of these processes is organized by that orchestra conductor, the pineal gland, using melatonin as a kind of baton.

It is probably best to wait for more research before taking melatonin. If you choose to use melatonin as a sleep aid, be sure to take the lowest effective dose about a half hour before bedtime. By the way, you'll probably find a number of different brands at your health-food store or pharmacy.

The synthetic form is preferable to that which is made from animal melatonin. And remember the problem with tryptophan; there may be harmful additives in some brands.

Finding the type of healing that works best for you may be a challenge. If you welcome everything that you learn along the journey, however, you may find that not only your insomnia is cured, but also that you have developed a new and more satisfying relationship to your health as a whole.

Chapter 7

The Ten Best Ways to Fall Asleep

A flock of sheep that leisurely pass by,
One after one; the sound of rain, and bees
murmuring; the fall of rivers, winds and seas,
Smooth fields, white sheets of water, and pure sky,
I have thought of all by turns and yet do lie
Sleepless! . . .
Come, blessed barrier between night and day
Dear mother of fresh thoughts and joyous health!

—Wordsworth

You've made a commitment to exercise, healthy diet, and meditation. You've gotten in touch with your own circadian rhythms and regularized your bedtime and wake time. You've taken steps to deal with some of the stress and frustrations in your life. But now it's actually time to go to bed. What do you do?

In this chapter, you'll find ten specific suggestions for making bedtime easier, more pleasant—and more likely to produce sleep. As with everything else in this book, use your own instincts about which ideas will work for you, and allow yourself to be inspired to come up with your own ideas.

1. *Make sure you have a comfortable bed.* A firm mattress and pillow are best—but make sure your pillow isn't too high, or your neck will be uncomfortable. Many people prefer natural fibers for their sheets and coverings, claiming that they're more conducive to comfortable temperatures.

What are your preferences for covers? Heavy? Light? Binding? Loose? See if you can make yourself as comfortable as possible, so that bed becomes an inviting place to be. If you sleep with a partner who has different preferences, work out a system whereby you can each have the type of sleep you prefer. It may take some doing, but be creative!

2. *Make sure your bedroom is conducive to sleep.* Is your room too light? Too noisy? Of a comfortable temperature? Provided with enough fresh air? These elements can make an enormous difference. Most people sleep better in a room that's a bit cooler at night than the temperature they'd prefer during the day. Fresh air is helpful for good respiration, which will help you sleep more deeply. Noise can disturb and agitate the nervous system, even while you're asleep, so if you can't block out traffic and other sounds, you might either invest in earplugs or play a tape of some soothing, even sound to fall asleep by, either a muffled "gray" sound or nature tapes of ocean or forest noises. Remember, too, that your bedroom is the last thing you see before you go to sleep at night. Provide yourself with soothing vistas that help you relax and feel at peace with yourself. Piles of unfinished work are probably the *least* helpful sight you could end the day with! But beyond just keeping work out of the bedroom, give some thought to what late-night sights would soothe your soul.

3. *Take a bath.* Baths not only help you relax, they help you make that body-temperature shift that can support your subjective sense of sleepiness. If you let your bath become a leisurely ritual, it can be a way of nurturing yourself, giving yourself one last treat so that the day feels full and you can say goodbye to it. Think about a bubble bath, bath pillows, a bath by candlelight or with a soothing cup of herb tea by your side. Aromatherapy can be a component of your bath (see the suggestions in Chapter 6), or you might combine your bath with a massage if you can find a willing partner.

4. *Drink a glass of warm milk or herb tea.* We've discussed why milk—rich in calcium and tryptophan—helps prepare you for sleep. The ritual of drinking something warm can also be a friendly way to reward yourself at the end of the day. Herb tea makes a good substitute for those trying to avoid dairy products.

5. *Do a relaxation exercise.* You've just finished your bath and are now lying on cool, freshly washed sheets. You see a beautiful Japanese print and a shelf of your favorite books from childhood, and contentedly you close your eyes. Now you're ready to relax. Breathe deeply and listen to a relaxation tape you've bought or made (see Chapter 6 for some ideas). Or listen to some peaceful music and allow your mind to wander. Either way, create a time when you can just savor the delicious sensations of your own body in your own space, free from obligations and worry. This can be a time you look forward to rather than one you dread.

6. *Do some light reading.* Maybe your idea of a bedtime treat is a good read—or maybe you're one of those "entrained" souls who can't fall asleep without reading at least a few pages. Try to choose a book that you can pick up and put down easily—a humorous work, a collection of short stories, even a favorite book from childhood that you're rereading. If you do a lot of "required reading" during the day, your nighttime reading might be a forbidden treat—what would that mean to you?

7. *Leave your worries outside the bedroom.* Some people engage in a ritual of writing their worries down in another room and then either burning the paper or storing it *outside* the bedroom. Other people imagine saying goodnight to their worries and shutting the door behind them. Still other people use visualizations of the kind described in Chapter 6. Whatever your preference, find a way to leave your worries somewhere else; keep the bedroom literally free of them.

8. *Make your last hour before bed as peaceful as possible.* Save intense conversations for another hour of the day. Avoid scary or suspenseful movies or TV shows. If you can get yourself away from television at least an hour before bedtime, that will also help ease your path to sleep; the flickering blue light of the television actually stimulates your nervous system, and falling asleep in front of the TV only means that you have to rouse yourself again to get to bed, breaking your sleep.

9. *Allow yourself to sleep—or, if your body chooses to stay awake, remain calmly mindful of yourself.* In other words, don't try to force or control anything, not even sleep. Just be aware of yourself and your body and let your mind go where it will. If you're tossing and turning, allow your body to do that as it prepares itself to rest. If your thoughts are racing madly, allow them to race—gently notice what they're doing, without judging or disapproving of yourself. Believe it or not, the fastest way to sleep is not to care when or even whether you get there. Just let your processes happen, remaining aware of them. Allowing the shift between restlessness and peacefulness can be a profound and powerful anti-insomnia device.

10. *Get up after half an hour or so, and do something that you like or need to do.* Decide that since you're giving yourself this waking time, you might as well do something pleasant with it. Find soothing treats for yourself that turn this late-night time into your own quiet time. Maybe at the moment you need that more than sleep.

Passing through insomnia can be a rocky journey indeed. At the end of the road, though, are sweet dreams and a peaceful night's rest. Enjoy!

INDEX